Suffering and Healing in America
An American doctor's view from outside

Suffering and Healing in America

An American doctor's view from outside

Raymond Downing

Foreword by
Ronald E. Pust

Radcliffe Publishing
Oxford • Seattle

Radcliffe Publishing Ltd
18 Marcham Road
Abingdon
Oxon OX14 1AA
United Kingdom

www.radcliffe-oxford.com
Electronic catalogue and worldwide online ordering facility.

British Library Cataloguing in Publication Data

A catalogue record for this book is available from the British Library.

ISBN-10 1 84619 130 0
ISBN-13 978 1 84619 130 5

Typeset by Egan Reid Ltd, Auckland, New Zealand
Printed and bound by Biddles Ltd, King's Lynn, Norfolk, UK

To my father

Contents

Foreword

It doesn't matter whether you are a provider or a consumer of health care, whether in the USA or outside, Dr. Ray Downing's latest book, *Suffering and Healing in America: An American doctor's view from outside*, continues to draw on his keenly reflective cultural insights to challenge us all.

As I write this, I am working in the most recent of Ray and Jan's North American settings of their learnings that he elicits in this book, the Navajo Area Indian Health Service. In 2003–2005, I joined Ray, Jan and others more experienced than I in East Africa in working with Kenyan physicians to launch the first family medicine residency education program in Kenya, at Moi University. There I saw Dr. Downing's most defining role in action, that of cultural broker at the interfaces between African and Western understandings, both medical and societal.

Born out of their earlier learnings in Appalachia and Africa described in Ray's autobiographic book, *The Wedding Goes on Without Us*,[1] the chapters in this new book also begin with concrete, personal stories, simple anecdotes that in most cultures are the beginning of profound learnings. Each of the sixteen short chapters apply this approach to the most foundational questions and paradigms (and sometimes, paradoxes) in health and healing.

Because they are so fundamental in human experience, each of these concepts could be employed in the explication of the healing enterprise in any culture. In fact, references to their roles in health of the varied members of the Hellenic pantheon are replete in this book. Here, however, Dr. Downing's manifest mandate is to help us dissect the cultural assumptions and values of our own American system (or non-system) from outside. Indeed, anthropologists confirm the wisdom of adages through the ages that exhort us to "first, know thyself", and of Robert Burns' supplication, "O, wad some Power the giftie gie us, to see ourselves as others see us". This book will help us see American health care in a worldwide context. And, if we are health care providers in America, whether we are family doctors (such as Ray and I are) or clinicians in any other of the myriad of American health professions, this book's lessons have much to teach us.

Not least of these lessons is cultural competence, recently recognized in USA medical and government agencies as a core component of quality health care. In fact, with this belated official mandate (and its accompanying money) to ensure cultural competency, it has become a cottage industry. Like other government mandates in US medical care, cultural competence will likely soon find its corporate niche in the US medical-industrial complex.

Dr. Downing, in contrast, has earned his stripes in cultural competency across two continents and three decades of clinical experience. His analyses, while carefully crafted and documented, come from the heart. And he does not wear these stripes ostentatiously, rarely offering advice or easy solutions. In this respect, he would agree with those who prefer the term cultural humility (Chapter 3 on Hubris). This is reflected in his preference for "learnings" over "teachings".

Nowhere among these chapters are Dr. Downing's insights more trenchant, or controversial, than in his exposition of *Chronic Disease* (Chapters 7 and 8) and *Prevention* (Chapters 12 and 13). Perhaps this is because in America both are medicalized toward life-long drug treatment. By contrast, in Africa, prevention is largely a societal, not a medical, responsibility. And suffering is borne, inherent in the meaning of life, rather than reflexively medicated.

In the USA there has been an explosion in the population of pharmaceuticals developed for the secondary prevention of cardiac and other chronic diseases. Witness also the debates about treating pre-hypertension[2] and pre-diabetes among other incipient neo-diseases. Closely akin is the direct marketing of prescription drugs to the general public, including new compounds for dubiously defined new diseases,[3,4] many of which are inherent in the human condition, such as occasional erectile dysfunction, heartburn, or restless legs. The pharmaceutical industry in the USA has created not only a pill for every ill but also, more recently in its disease-mongering,[5] an ill for every pill.

Dr. Downing does not reject these trends out-of-hand, but subjects them to that newest of paradigms in Western health care - evidence-based medicine. Pointing out the typically astonishingly high NNT (number needed to treat, i.e., number of patients treated to produce the targeted outcome for *one* person), he shows that America's societal willingness to invest in these medical treatments ultimately reflects the American culture. America has money and science; but we may have abandoned the spiritual and social context of our lives, and deaths. In Africa, and in many other places on our planet, it is quite the opposite. I invite you to explore these contrasts with Dr. Ray Downing.

Ronald E. Pust MD
Professor of Family and Community Medicine and of Public Health
University of Arizona College of Medicine
Tucson, Arizona
rpust@u.arizona.edu
July 2006

References

1 Downing R (2002) *The Wedding Goes on Without Us, including Bury Me Naked.* Jacaranda Designs, Nairobi.

2 Mitka M (2006) Experts ponder treating prehypertension. *JAMA.* **295:** 2125–6.

3 Moynihan R and Cassels A (2005) *Selling Sickness: How the World's Biggest Pharmaceutical Companies are Turning us all into Patients.* Nation Books, New York, NY.

4 Dyer O (2006) Disease awareness campaigns turn healthy people into patients. *BMJ.* **332:** 871.

5 Moynihan R and Henry D (2006) The fight against disease-mongering: generating knowledge for action. *PloS Medicine.* 3 (No. 4, April). Much of this issue of this peer-reviewed journal, which does not accept advertising, is devoted to this topic. Available online at: http://medicine.plosjournals.org

Preface

I did not begin writing this book with a well-developed theory of American medicine in mind. I began instead with feelings and reactions to my own occupation, perceptions that had been growing as I moved and read. I had been trained in America and had worked for seven years in America, but then I left home to work in Africa in 1985. While there, I began to explore the essence of medicine and during May and June of 1996, I wrote the first drafts of about half of the following essays. The impetus then was to prepare for a year-long research and teaching sabbatical at the University of Tennessee Department of Family Medicine in Knoxville, the same place I had trained. After returning to Kenya, I wrote several more chapters – often when a medical student visiting from the US or a news story would remind me how different Western medicine was from what I had been practicing in Africa for over a decade. Then I came home again in 2001, this time to work seeing patients – and experienced the shock of everything I had been writing about.

Good writing may be a private activity; good thinking rarely is. My wife Jan, also a doctor, has lived every one of these essays with me. Dr Ron Pust has been a most perceptive critic and cheerleader since these essays were in their infancy. Dr Cathleen Morrow kindly reviewed the entire manuscript at short notice, and the Radcliffe staff have been exemplary in bringing this book to print. I am grateful also to the Graduate School of Medicine in Knoxville for giving me the opportunity to begin developing these thoughts, and to the many faculty members there who critiqued early drafts. I am particularly grateful to the chairman, Dr Greg Blake, who opened my mind to this approach. I was ready to spend my sabbatical teaching about travel medicine, but he asked me the larger question: what did my African experience have to say about American healthcare? This book is my response.

Raymond Downing
July 2006

About the author

Raymond Downing is an American medical doctor who has spent more of his professional life working in Africa than in the US. His first book, *The Wedding Goes on Without Us*, records the story of his journey from working for seven years among poor people in the US to working for 15 years in three African countries: Sudan, Tanzania, and Kenya. It is also the story of his growing understanding of African healing wisdom, and is the foundation for the perspective in his next two books. The second book, *As They See It*, tells the story of the development of the discourse on AIDS in Africa. Yet although the subject matter is AIDS, the African reflections come with an invitation to look beyond the specific disease being examined. AIDS is providing the world with an opportunity to see how Africans view health and disease generally.

On returning to the US in 2001 to work for three years on the Navajo Indian Reservation for the US Indian Health Service, he continued some ongoing reflections and contrasts between healthcare in the US and Africa. The current book is the result.

Raymond Downing is married to Dr Janice Armstrong and they have two grown children, Elizabeth and Timothy. He and his wife both work for the Department of Family Medicine, Moi University School of Medicine, Eldoret, Kenya.

CHAPTER ONE

Introduction

My father lived a good long life but never learned to swallow pills. He was in other respects an exemplary American: an Eagle Scout, a chemical engineer, a World War II veteran. He was a logical man who liked things planned, organized, and written down; a scientist – and his embracing of science included the science of medicine. His wife had several surgical operations; his two daughters both became nurses, his son a doctor who married a doctor. He found medicine fascinating.

At the end of his life, when my sister brought him to the hospital with his heart attack at age 85, she could not get him to settle down and go to sleep. He was interested in everything going on around him in the emergency room, and didn't want to miss anything. His interest, however, had nothing to do with his own life and impending death, for those were matters he had settled long before. He had passed the Biblical 'threescore years and ten' and 'by reason of strength,' he even passed the fourscore. He was not expecting from medicine any extension to his life or even improvement; it simply fascinated him the same way a hardware store did.

That hospitalization was his only one – except for a childhood tonsillectomy back when they were in fashion. He had no more surgery and took no regular medications until after he passed 80. Then he was told he had diabetes and chewed some pills for a while – and later still chewed some other pills that were supposed to help his failing memory. When, a few days after his heart attack, he had a massive stroke, there was no struggle for my sisters and I to decide to discontinue IV fluids; we knew it was what he would have wanted. He had instructed us to cremate him after he died, not for any family or religious reasons but simply because he wanted to minimize funeral expenses – America's final medical care, the part we never study for cost-effectiveness.

My father never learned to swallow pills: a most profound if unconscious rebellion against modern medical care. The first requirement of being a patient is being able to swallow pills – and our healthcare system tells us that we are all patients now, even we who are healthy. We are told we can remain that way by taking pills and when we get sick, pills will help us get better. Most of us accept this patient role because we trust what our healthcare system tells us – for after all, we believe, Western healthcare, and American particularly, is the best in the world.

This may be true regarding technology: virtually all Nobel prize winners in medicine have been European or American. It is of course more debatable whether the American healthcare *system* is the world's best, and Europe provides several alternative delivery systems.[1] However, deeper than technological medicine *or* the system which delivers it are the fundamental matters of health, suffering, healing, and prevention. These are the matters my father refused to delegate to the healthcare system; these are the matters this book addresses.

People in all cultures and throughout history have confronted life and death, mostly without Western healthcare. This experience has, not surprisingly, resulted in some assumptions about suffering and healing: that suffering is inevitable, that healing is spiritual, and that both are a mystery. Modern Western healthcare has rightly challenged some of these assumptions with its technological advances that have made some of the suffering and death 'unnecessary.' However, these 'miracles' can upstage the wisdom about suffering and healing that history and other cultures have on offer. Paradoxically, the more we can cure and relieve pain, the less we understand about suffering and healing.

However, advanced technology in healthcare is not incompatible with traditional wisdom. Many Third World countries utilize Western medical technology without losing their traditional understandings of suffering and healing, just as my father did. Though balancing the two can be difficult, some combination is better than either alone. Perhaps we need the 'gospel' of technological medicine preached back to us by those who have adopted it without abandoning their own wisdom. This book is one such attempt, looking at Western healthcare, including its technology, from an 'outside' perspective: outside Western paradigms, and sometimes outside the 20th century. My goal is to show how our own healthcare system is suffering – and, by implication, how it might be healed.

Healthcare is about people and this book is full of stories about people who faced illness and their healthcare system. Each story introduces or illustrates the 'issue' or 'point' about modern Western healthcare contained in that chapter, and each chapter could stand alone. Because of this, the reader may lose the overall argument of the book in the details of the issues. To guard against getting lost, the following is a concise development of the book's central thesis.

Health

We sometimes call the entire enterprise of Western medicine a 'healthcare system' but of course, it is really a disease care system. We use the broader term 'healthcare' because we want to produce and preserve health, and our assumption is that eliminating or avoiding disease ensures health. It may, but of course health is far more than the mere absence of disease, in the same way that peace is more than the absence of war. Health literally means wholeness and is included in the Hebrew concept 'shalom,' usually translated as peace. A true healthcare system would have to include the government, religion, and culture of a people – and this is the foundation of the claim in Chapter 2, not original with me, that health is not primarily a medical matter.

However, we have a paradigm of medical care (Chapter 3) which limits itself to the mechanics of disease and assumes that health is regained by medicines and surgery. The system admits the need for sanitation, proper nutrition, appropriate 'lifestyle' choices, and even spiritual harmony for good health but none of these is the primary business of the healthcare system. Medicine and surgery are, and are offered – often quite successfully – for maintenance as well as repair of health.

It is, in fact, the remarkable success of Western medical care which has led to our hubris (Chapter 4), our presumption that by pursuing our scientific paradigm further, we can control life and disease and even death. This hubris leads in turn to bizarre ethical dilemmas (Chapter 5) which, when they become lawsuits, we cannot ignore. As long as the foundation of our system is disease elimination by technology, this cascade of success leading to hubris leading to ethical and legal dilemmas will continue.

Suffering

To free ourselves from these dilemmas, we need to go back to the beginning, to health. If health is wholeness, then any challenge to that wholeness – pain, disease, war, poverty or any other affliction – will result in suffering (Chapter 6). The scientific disease elimination paradigm seeks to eliminate this suffering, which it equates with affliction. But suffering literally refers to how we bear the affliction, not the affliction itself. Western medicine has done well in helping to reduce disease affliction, but it does us a disservice when it tries also to reduce our suffering, our ability to carry the affliction it cannot eliminate.

Things get more complicated when we consider chronic disease (Chapters 7 and 8), one of the principal causes of suffering in Western countries. These are conditions which modern medicine has not been able to eliminate but only 'manage' – albeit often quite successfully. The consequence, however, is that people with chronic diseases become permanent patients, dependent on the medical system. That system works to reduce their affliction, but the continued presence of their disease is a continuing challenge to their wholeness and therefore a continued source of suffering. Modern medicine offers dependence on itself to reduce this suffering, when what the patient really needs is an enhancement of the ability to suffer, or carry the affliction.

Healing

What modern medicine offers is treatment, not healing (Chapter 9). Treatment may play a part in healing, but healing involves spiritual and cultural dimensions, such as enhancing the ability to suffer, which are beyond the scope of technological disease elimination (Chapter 10). Unfortunately, the more effective the technology becomes, the more the culture loses its understanding of healing. Family medicine was in part an attempt by the medical system itself to recover and preserve the healing arts of our culture (Chapter 11). One role originally envisioned for family medicine was coordinator of technology to enhance healing. However, that part of the family medicine movement is being threatened by other priorities of the healthcare system; a more prominent role today is gate-keeper for the technological disease elimination system. And while the patients are waiting at the gate, we offer medicalized prevention.

Prevention

Prevention is common sense and our healthcare system openly advocates prevention. However, our emphases in prevention lack some of that common sense. The healthcare system offers us what it knows best: secondary prevention – screening tests to diagnose disease early and medicines to manage 'risk factors' (Chapter 12). Because of the authority and success of our system in eliminating disease, we embrace this form of prevention. That is sensible. What makes less sense is gradually coming to equate prevention with early diagnosis or medical management of risk factors.

The best form of prevention, of course, is primary prevention – keeping a disease from happening in the first place. But as noted above, this kind of prevention is the business of society and culture, more than the healthcare system. Nevertheless, the system does have some responsibility in public policy (Chapter 13) and should never let secondary prevention overshadow primary prevention.

Culture

If our healthcare system is, as I have suggested, both very effective and very limited, with the successes themselves upstaging the deficiencies, what can be done to correct the problems without losing the benefits? Is there any hope? There is, and paradoxically it comes from contact with poorer societies that practice Western healthcare, societies that do not have our hubris and cannot afford to let go of their own indigenous healing systems. The first effect of contact with these other cultures is to see our own system anew (Chapter 14).

When we look at ourselves from outside, we can see more clearly our own wealth as well as our waste, our excellence and our extremes, our successes, and our silliness. And then, when we keep looking, we may even begin to ask of those other cultures how they do things, and if there is anything we can learn from them (Chapter 15).

And finally, if we can find a way to transform our hubris into humility, we may be ready to listen to our own poor patients (Chapter 16). Or perhaps, listening to our poor patients may be a route to humility.

HEALTH

CHAPTER TWO

Health

'Why did you say healing isn't your real work?' . . . Damfo spoke first: 'We heal people, individuals. That's part of our work. But it isn't all. It isn't even the greater part of it. It's just a part. The whole of it concerns . . .' the effort to find a word threatened to exasperate him, but he breathed deep, smiled, and said with an air of giving up, '. . . wholeness.'

Ayi Kwei Armah, *The Healers*

First, a story from Tanzania

They brought him in during the week before Easter: a young man, married, with small children, who'd just had half his face blown away by an explosion in a gold mine. Another doctor at our hospital cleaned him up the best he could when he arrived. His right eye was gone, his cheek open, his palate fractured, and his left eye beyond repair.

Besides giving him antibiotics, the only thing we could do was change the dressing every day. We'd give something to lessen the pain, peel off the bandages, and wash out the pus that was developing. Each day we cut off a little more dead tissue and each day we removed some more dirt embedded in his brain behind the eye socket. By this time he had florid meningitis and spinal fluid leaked continuously from his right ear.

Why, then, was he still awake and alert, talking, and drinking water? There was, it seemed, some hope for him to survive – if he could get to a hospital big enough to provide reconstructive surgery. His family was ready to take him a couple days after admission, but that would mean traveling on the Easter holidays and we were afraid he'd be neglected if he arrived at another hospital on a holiday. Wait till the Tuesday after Easter, we suggested.

Tuesday got changed to Thursday, and then Friday. Another weekend approached. Please be sure to take him on Friday, I pleaded with the family. Yes, yes, they assured me.

But on Friday a new hope appeared. A priest had been admitted a few days before following an automobile accident. He had a broken shoulder blade, but otherwise was fine. The bishop had decided to send the diocese airplane to pick him up on Saturday and bring him to one of Tanzania's biggest referral hospitals. When the injured miner found out, his family asked if he could go as well. The priest was willing, assuming the pilot agreed. Would I discuss it with the pilot?

Saturday morning. The plane was due to arrive between 8 and 9. At 9.30, new developments: some other people wanted rides and the plane would be delayed until 11.00. I was going out to another village that morning and had to leave by 10.00. I wrote a referral letter, discharged the miner, and signed out to two other doctors, fearful that something would go wrong and the miner would be delayed another day. I was beginning, too, to be frustrated because the one who needed the transfer urgently had no guarantee of a ride and the one who had access to the plane could have been treated adequately at our hospital.

I got back at 5.30. The miner had not gone on the plane – something about an unpressurized cabin being dangerous to him – but because he had already been discharged he was not getting antibiotics or dressing changes. He finally left early Sunday morning, without IVs, antibiotics or even a fresh dressing, for the 14-hour Land Rover trip across the Serengeti Plains.

Several days later I got word that he was dead.

What is it about this story that affects you most? Is it that we had no surgical team or equipment to give this man a chance to live? That is indeed unfortunate and, seen through American medical eyes, tragic. We know that if this accident had happened in America, he would at least have had a chance to live. It is one of the 'if onlys' we run into every day in practicing medicine in Africa.

But lack of readily available technology and expertise is not the most important difference from the American healthcare system, at least as I see it. There are plenty of other 'if onlys.' For example . . .

The gold mine that this man worked in was one of several dozen hand-dug holes, each a hundred or more feet deep, each about as wide as a pit latrine. The miners blasted the rock at the bottom with dynamite charges, then removed the loose pieces by passing them in trays hand to hand up a chain of people from the bottom of the mine to the surface. There was no OSHA to ensure – or even suggest – safety precautions. There were no hard hats at the mine, no first aid station, no telephone or radio communication with a rescue squad, and no ambulance. The only technology present, other than the dynamite, was a diesel pump to remove water from the mines. Even before the accident, our miner had two strikes against him.

But he did not die at the bottom of his mine where the accident occurred, and his friends were able to extract him, find a vehicle, and transport him to our hospital. That was a three-hour journey at least, if the roads were dry. The first half hour was up a steep, rocky road to the top of an escarpment, traveling at no more than five miles per hour. None of the roads between the mine and our hospital was paved.

It is true that he passed the government district hospital on the way to our mission hospital. It was well known that government hospitals had so little funding that they usually had no medicines or surgical supplies. The decision to bypass one hospital with a dangerously ill patient was an intelligent one.

The difficulties of transport did not end when he arrived at our hospital. In the end it was lack of transport, not lack of medical technology, that defeated him. Transportation – plenty of it, and available to anyone critically ill – is a vital part of the American healthcare system. We saw that particularly clearly in our hospital in Tanzania, where it was lacking not just for our miner but for all of our patients.

Our hospital was the only place within a 30-mile radius able to offer major surgery and blood transfusions, and we served a population of about 100 000 people. We were not in a city and the population was relatively evenly distributed. I decided to look at where our patients came from, especially those requiring services not available in clinics or smaller hospitals. I chose caesarean sections and blood transfusions for children with severe anemia from malaria. I found that the rate of these procedures was much higher for women and children living close to the hospital, and was inversely related to distance.[1] That is, the farther a village was from the hospital, the fewer people from that village came for procedures they could get nowhere else. And the gradient dropped sharply about 10 miles away from the hospital: the distance someone could comfortably come by foot or bicycle.

In other words, a principal determinant of obtaining healthcare technology in Tanzania is not the availability of that technology, but the availability of transportation to get to it. When we didn't have it, we saw how much transportation is a part of any healthcare system.[2] So are safety precautions, nationwide compulsory education, widespread vaccinations, a healthy economy – and, of course, pipes.

Pipes may, in fact, be the most important part of America's healthcare system, especially when compared with Third World healthcare systems. Almost every American can get relatively clean water out of a pipe in or very near home. Most Americans deposit their stool in toilets connected to pipes which carry the refuse to treatments plants. Rarely, these systems of pipes malfunction, resulting in an outbreak of diarrhea in a community. Such an outbreak is 'reportable,' and the community is swamped with epidemiologists, public health officers, chlorine, and portable chemical johns.

Compare this with a typical rural African community. Some villages have wells in the center of town with hand pumps, supplying water for people bucket by bucket only five or 10 minutes from home. Other villages are less fortunate and the women need to walk 15 or 20 minutes to the nearest stream or spring to carry back one five-gallon bucket of water. In the dry season, the distance may be 45 minutes one way. The fortunate homes usually have pit latrines with mud walls and a grass roof but some people, poorer or less educated or nomadic, use no latrines at all.

These villages, the ones with few latrines and water sources far away, do not have 'outbreaks' of diarrhea; they have endemic diarrhea, affecting especially the children. One episode of diarrhea rarely kills, but chronic or recurrent diarrhea leads to dehydration, decreased appetite, undernutrition, and susceptibility to other diseases. And, commonly, death. In our hospital in Tanzania, three-fourths of the deaths were of children.

The American healthcare system has clearly succeeded in keeping most of America's children alive. The infant mortality rate is about one-tenth that of many African countries. The system can be proud – but congratulations go not to the surgeons and scanners but to the pipes.[3]

So, the first lesson from Africa about our healthcare system is that health is not primarily a medical matter.[4] People in our society may not all be healthy, but in comparison with the Third World – using gross indicators such as total death rates and infant and maternal mortality rates – we are far better off. And the reasons are social and economic much more than medical.

Nevertheless, there are major differences between the medical systems of Third World countries and those of America and other Western countries. First of all, traditional healers (called 'witch doctors' in the past) still play a major role in healthcare. But even the Western parts of the medical systems are different, though *the difference is more in quantity than in quality*. That, at least, is my opinion and brings us to the crux of what we can learn when seeing our own medical system from the point of view of its 'offspring' in Third World countries.

In America we pride ourselves on having a very high standard of medical care. To us, that standard involves both quantity and quality. We have not only *more* diagnostic tests and therapeutics than some other societies, but also *better* ones. After all, our products are not washing machines or hedge clippers but technology that directly affects human life – and we take that seriously. To maintain our standard we will cut no corners. Our motto might be a combination of 'Only The Best' with 'More Is Better.'

But is that the essence of a high standard? Let's look at a simple procedure readily available in both America and the Third World: the lumbar puncture – obtaining a small amount of spinal fluid for analysis by inserting a needle into a person's back. Undoubtedly most American laboratories can do far more sophisticated analysis on the spinal fluid than most African labs, though the basic tests are universally available. But let's look just at the process of *getting* the fluid. In America this involves a several hundred dollar disposable kit with everything you need to clean and anesthetize the skin, measure the pressure, and collect the fluid. In Africa we cleanse the skin, obtain the fluid from children with a disposable 21-gauge needle (the same kind we use for drawing blood and giving injections), then collect it in a clean recycled medicine bottle. For adults, we use specially made spinal needles, if we have them. In both places we get fluid without harm to the patient – but in America we use more equipment and the cost is higher. Does that represent a better, or higher, standard?[5]

Before answering – that is, before trying to either defend American medicine or rail against its excesses – let's consider more carefully one implication of such high quality and quantity: cost. That healthcare costs are spiraling upwards is undisputed. That was a principal reason for the attempted US healthcare reforms of 1993–94, and for managed care. Several culprits were identified: the technology itself, the insurance companies, the increasing government regulation and paperwork, the malpractice game, physician fees, drug company profits, and so on. From the perspective of people who work with limited resources, these are all sink-holes, all bottomless pits with insatiable appetites. But several – technology, drug company research, and probably physician reimbursement – are related to our high standard of medical care.

Yet, as we saw at the beginning, these are not the main reasons why Americans are as healthy as they are; they are not the major factors in preventing disease or promoting health. None is as important as pipes or good roads or basic education or vaccinations in producing a healthy population. Of course, my 80-year-old mother could not have gotten her knee joint replacement in Tanzania, and of course, I'm glad she got it in Massachusetts. But she could have gotten a lumbar puncture in Tanzania were she to need it, and she could get fully effective treatment for many common conditions there. Our high standard has apparently not stopped to look at itself, to seriously consider the effect of quality on health, or the effect of quantity on quality. To maintain a high medical standard, is it necessary to have unlimited quality, unlimited quantity . . . and unlimited cost?

But spiraling costs were not the only impetus for healthcare reform in 1993–94. A major irony in our system of unlimited medical care is how limited is its availability. Acute life-saving care may be theoretically available to everyone but ongoing elective care clearly is not. Substantial segments of our population are unserved or under-served (my Freudian spell-check reads that last word as 'undeserved').

This irony of a system with apparently unlimited quality and quantity, at the expense of limited availability, was more than matched by the irony of reform efforts which tried to reduce the costs and, at the same time, expand coverage of this same unlimited system. The economic sleight-of-hand involved apparently fooled no one. We could not offer the same costly healthcare to

13

more people and have it cost less. Instead, we settled for government and insurance companies breathing down our necks asking us to justify certain costs, while we continue to use $100 lumbar puncture sets which no one questions, and homeless men in Washington DC sleep on steam grates in the winter while their legs rot off.

Ironically, it may be the view from outside which gives us hope. That view tells us that our healthcare system is very good, but not primarily because of our medical technology. It tells us that it is possible to provide quality medical care without always relying on expensive high-level technology. And that view can also tell us something about practicing medicine among needy, under-served people, a topic requiring its own chapter (16). The view from outside suggests that we physicians should be the first to reform our own system, and it gives us some insight about how to do that.

CHAPTER THREE

Paradigms

I saw the weakness of the whites. It wasn't military at all. It was a weakness of the spirit, the soul. The whites are not on friendly terms with the surrounding universe. Between them and the universe there is real hostility. Take the forest here. If they stay long in the forest, they die. Either they cut down the forest and kill it, or it kills them. They can't live with it.

Ayi Kwei Armah, *The Healers*

A paradigm is a grand pattern or model, often of the way some great enterprise is carried out. It's an oft-used word today, especially in the face of major political and social changes. People who work in the Third World refer to 'paradigm shifts' in mission or development. This is no mere change in theory about how to do something; a paradigm shift is a fundamental change in the assumptions of what is worth doing and why, as well as how to do it.

A paradigm is hard to recognize from 'inside.' Paradigms are like air: we never think about air until its composition changes drastically or we don't have it at all. Likewise with any great enterprise, we are able to fully describe the paradigm underlying it only when it has been replaced by a new perspective. It is very difficult to articulate the assumptions underlying our own enterprise, precisely because those assumptions are so widely shared but rarely stated. Earthbound people spend little time talking about the need to breathe air, though city dwellers may complain about its poor quality. Astronauts, on the other hand, are constantly aware of their need for air.

Both the technology and organization of American healthcare are changing fast. We will look at some of these changes and their underlying paradigms in Chapter 7. However, I do not think the American healthcare system is undergoing a *fundamental* paradigm shift. That happened over a century ago when we adopted biomedical scientific medicine. All the current debates and changes seem firmly anchored in our present underlying assumptions, or paradigm. I think there is value in trying to describe that paradigm – with some help from 'the view from outside' – in order to see our roots more clearly. Then we will be in a better position to see if it still resonates with reality.

Before using the paradigms of other times and places to see ourselves more clearly, however, we can first look at how we describe ourselves, especially in relation to alternative healing paradigms in our own society. Medical textbooks speak of the 'scientific methods and principles' underlying our approach to medicine, which should be characterized by 'objectivity,' leading to the 'prevention and cure of disease and the relief of suffering.'[1] In other words, we want to understand where disease comes from and get rid of it by whatever method actually works. Of course. But what this also says is that we are not committed to *one* preconceived notion of where all disease comes from (for example, evil spirits), nor to one method of treatment (for example, exorcism). We are, however, committed to one method of investigation: verifiable science.

But the commitment to a single, unitary theory of disease and therapy is the characteristic of many medical paradigms. Chiropractic is a good example, viewing disease as emanating from disorders of the spinal column, and therefore treatment as manipulation of the spinal column. At best, Western medicine views this approach as limited and temporary; at worst, as quackery. Similarly with homeopathy, 'a system of medical treatment based on the theory that certain diseases can be cured by giving very small doses of drugs which in a healthy person and in large doses would produce symptoms like those of the disease.'[2] At best, harmless. At worst, more quackery.

But if we step back and look more dispassionately at these other paradigms, are they really so foreign to us? Doesn't *some* disease result from bony pressure on spinal nerves? Doesn't chiropractic manipulation sometimes give at least as much temporary relief as our treatment for back pain? And doesn't our practice of vaccination to prevent disease fit almost exactly into the homeopathic paradigm? In other words, our problem with chiropractic and homeopathy is not the paradigm itself, but the attempt to apply it to all disease. Our 'scientific' paradigm is built on verifiable pragmatism and includes such disparate approaches to therapy as drugs, surgery, vaccinations, physical therapy, counseling – as long as they can be 'proven' to work.

This scientific paradigm of medicine is actually a blending of two streams of thought. The Enlightenment contributed the scientific approach, but the contribution was to an existing paradigm of medicine: allopathy. This was the 'orthodox' paradigm of the 19th century, named by the sectarian homeopaths[3] who saw them treating 'by remedies that produce effects different from or opposite to those produced by the disease.'[4] That seemed to work more often than homeopathy. Aspirin lowers body temperature when it's high; antihypertensives lower blood pressure, even when it isn't high. Insulin lowers blood sugar. And so forth. The scientific approach found far more resonance with allopathy than with homeopathy.

Today we no longer talk about a remedy as needing to produce the opposite effect to the disease, but we have not wholly abandoned our allopathic roots. There is implied in allopathy the sense of clobbering a disease into submission, of reversing what the disease has done, of controlling the problem with remedies – sentiments we appreciate. This approach is quite different from that implicit in homeopathy, and explicit in naturopathy, to only work together with natural healing processes. These are paradigmatic differences and that's where we part company. We have no quarrel with the immune system fighting infection, but we'll 'help' it with antibiotics whenever we can. Sun may be fine for acne, but tetracycline works better. If we only 'help nature take its course' then we haven't done anything to 'fight disease,' which our paradigm tells us we must do.

To summarize so far: our 'modern' or 'Western' paradigm of healthcare is 'a science of the physical, with a primary orientation toward the identification and eradication of empirically confirmed disease.'[5] We do not have a single unifying concept of the origin of disease. Some, we say, is due to the 'intrusion' of outside factors (infections); some is inherited from our ancestors (genetic disease); some is from body parts wearing out (degenerative diseases); some is 'accidental.' Our paradigm can accept the therapies of other paradigms if their efficacies can be 'empirically confirmed.'

Now let's step back a bit from our own society and its history of conflicting paradigms, and consider the view from outside. The medical anthropologist J. M. Janzen says that 'using a broad perspective, ideas at the basis of most of the world's health and medical systems may be divided between those that explain causation (of health and disease) by a theory of **balance** and those that explain it by a theory of **intrusion**.'[6]

This statement applies historically as well as geographically. Galen's humoral theory is an example. This paradigm of medicine held sway in Europe for almost 1500 years and was widely accepted in our country at the time of independence. It was based on the Hippocratic belief that there were four humors in our bodies: blood, mucus or phlegm, yellow bile, and black bile. They needed to be in balance to remain healthy; an excess or 'agitation' of one over the others caused disease. Therapy was to reduce the one in excess by, for example, bleeding or purging.

Likewise traditional Chinese medicine is based on the need for balance between the forces of Yin (structure, substance, etc.) and Yang (action, expansion, etc.) to maintain health. Ayurvedic medicine, still practiced in India, sees health as 'a balance of humors, vital breaths, heat and cold', etc. and seeks 'the harmony of multiple aspects of life.' Some of the broadest concepts of balance are in North American Indian health paradigms, seeking balance with the entire cosmos to maintain health, with therapy being geared to restore a person 'to his appropriate position in the universe.'[7]

Traditional African understandings of health and disease also involve balance or, as Africans might call it, relationship. A healthy people is a people in right relationship with God and each other. Disease means that some relationship is broken (out of balance) and the underlying question for Africans who are sick is not 'how did I get sick?' or even 'what do I have?' but 'why am I sick?' and 'which relationship is broken?'. Restoring the relationship restores health.

This brief overview is not meant to suggest that all traditional paradigms are the same, rooted in the balance theory. They are not. But it does seem apparent that many cultures through world history have sensed that health is somehow related to balance and harmony – whether within the body or within a society or in the whole universe – and disease to imbalance. The other paradigm, **intrusion,** is also widespread in traditional societies, especially as it includes not just the intrusion of germs and invading armies but also of evil spirits. Some healthcare paradigms have elements of both theories intertwined – or perhaps we should say, held in balance.

Returning to our own Western, scientific healthcare paradigm, it appears once again that we are eclectic and have within our system elements of both intrusion and balance. We understand intrusion immediately: bacteria and viruses intrude, bullets and knives intrude, cigarette smoke or radiation intrudes to induce cancers, even events or people intrude to make us anxious or depressed. Our allopathic 'clobbering a disease into submission' with surgery or powerful drugs fits this paradigm.

But we also believe in balance. A person with goiter can have too much thyroid hormone or not enough thyroid hormone; our task is not to get rid of thyroid hormone, but to bring it back into balance. A person with allergy or autoimmune disease has an overactive immune system; our job is not to eliminate it, but to bring it back into balance. Much of psychiatry and family therapy is trying to restore balance to an unbalanced psyche or family.

Nevertheless, despite our using both balance and intrusion theories, we are far more familiar and comfortable with intrusion.[8] Most of the time we see disease as intrusion, not imbalance, and most of our therapies are very intrusive. Even when we seek to restore balance, we often do so with powerful drugs (steroids in autoimmune disease) or surgery (thyroidectomy). Our way of trying to restore balance is by *controlling* the imbalance.

Naturally, our view of imbalance rarely extends beyond the body, though family medicine has at least widened the scope to the nuclear family.[9] We may grant that imbalance in a society, or ecological imbalance, can indirectly result in disease, but our paradigm does not attempt therapy for those imbalances. We don't even try to imagine the effects of cosmic imbalance on health, because we don't know what cosmic imbalance is.

And we don't apologize for under-emphasizing balance. After all, the 'success rate' using our paradigm has been pretty good; excellent, in fact. No other paradigm has consistently eliminated infectious diseases, restored hormonal imbalances, cured cancers, brought back severely traumatized people from the brink of death . . .

No, and people of other paradigms appreciate our successes; there are 'Western' hospitals all over the world. But, oddly, those hospitals have not supplanted all other paradigms, have not even suppressed them, it seems. I was riding with a young fellow in Tanzania one day and I asked him where he'd go if he got malaria. To our hospital, he said. What about jaundice? To the local healer. Anemia? Our hospital, for a transfusion. A broken bone? The local bone-setter. That 19-year-old boy had a well worked out triage system based on symptoms and his knowledge of what herbalists and bone-setters could successfully treat or, in the case of hepatitis, what he knew we couldn't treat. His system offered him things we couldn't.

But it isn't just herbs and skilled bone-setters. His *paradigm* offered him things our paradigm doesn't. His paradigm, by addressing the question uppermost in his mind – *why* he was sick – dealt with his disease in ways that allowed him to begin to restore the imbalances in his life or family or village. Africans know that our paradigm ultimately only deals with symptoms. Our paradigm's answer to the 'broader picture' in Africa is public health, and that does scratch a bit deeper. But we would never attempt to deal with spiritual questions. Yet to most traditional Africans, all questions of health and disease, all questions of life, are spiritual questions.

To say it another way, our paradigm consciously limits itself to the mechanics of disease – and that can be done effectively using an intrusion theory of causation and therapy. Our paradigm has been able to control many diseases without bothering to find out *why* they occur, but simply *how*. We have not involved ourselves in matters of balance in a community – or in the universe – because our therapeutic intrusions into the body or nuclear family are 'effective.' We don't need to go any deeper. What we do works well enough so that, in our paradigm, we doctors are the end of the line – even when we don't want to be.

And that's where the problems begin. We doctors – especially family physicians – usually know our limitations and we know that physicians cannot cure all disease. Though we enjoy relating to patients and trying to relieve suffering, we resent the expectation that we ought to cure everything, and that if something goes wrong, it's our fault. We want to take out a full page newspaper ad and proclaim WE ARE NOT GODS. The malpractice industry posits for us deity that we don't want, then sues us based on the failure to perform as gods.

But in our paradigm, there is nothing to appeal to beyond us. Our successes have raised expectations (if we can cure pneumonia and appendicitis, why not AIDS and cancer?), expectations we cannot fill, and our paradigm offers no alternative treatment or explanation. We can say, 'Some day science may find a cure for conditions like yours,' but that offers no hope for the one suffering. We cannot say, 'You are out of balance in your community, or in your cosmos, and this is what you must do to get back in balance.' We don't believe this, nor do our patients; it's not part of our commonly agreed paradigm.

We may not want to admit it, but the malpractice industry has found the Achilles heel of our paradigm and has shamelessly exploited it. We do not deal with the grander questions of why people get sick, of disturbed relationships between people and their environment and God, of imbalance in the cosmos. When we cannot heal, when something goes wrong, we are the end of the line.

How different from our experience in Africa. There we work in a hospital built on the Western scientific paradigm, but we work with people always aware of the larger questions. When someone dies unexpectedly, when something goes wrong or even when we make a mistake, patients and their families do not get angry. They do not feel let down by the medical system. They thank us for what we've done, knowing that we are only God's servants, knowing that we do not control awesome matters like life and death, knowing that our contribution is only a part of the attempt to restore balance.

Consider this incident. I have never liked being on call, though dramatic situations sometimes overcome the distaste. The reason for being called just before midnight on this occasion, however, did not seem dramatic and I was irritated. One of the nurses at our hospital in Kenya had given birth earlier that day and now her baby wasn't nursing well. The birth had been uneventful, the baby had no fever, his exam was normal; he just wasn't nursing well.

My technique for these kind of calls was to wake up enough to make a good decision, but not so much that I'd have trouble getting back to sleep. It could be a tough balancing act, trying to wake up just enough to decide what was dramatic, so that I could decide whether or not to wake up more. This case was typical: the baby just didn't look sick, but I knew that not nursing could be a symptom of something serious. I had only two choices – start the baby on antibiotics or do nothing – and I wanted to decide and go back to bed. I couldn't decide.

Since the mom was a nurse, I asked her opinion. Well, she thought, the baby wasn't *that* sick (though he was sick enough for her to wake me up, I reflected later) and giving antibiotics meant injections for the poor little fellow . . . Aw, let's just watch him tonight and see how he is in the morning. Good idea, I agreed. And I went back to sleep.

The next morning I told the situation to my wife, who is a pediatrician. She wondered that I hadn't been called back to see the baby and went directly to the hospital to see him. He looked awful; she started him on the antibiotics I should have given the night before. It was too late. Four hours later he was dead.

The mom was devastated. Within 24 hours the struggle and joy of birth had been turned upside down. She'd had nine months to prepare for his life and just a few hours to prepare for his death – a death, I was well aware, I might have been able to prevent. Whenever something bad happens, I review my actions, to see if I would do anything different if it came up again. Most of the time I can defend, to myself at least, what I did. But this time I could not. There was enough evidence at the time to consider a diagnosis of sepsis and begin proper treatment. I considered the diagnosis, but did not begin the treatment. I was wrong.

A few hours after the death, the baby's dad approached me, not as doctor but as custodian of the mission vehicle. Could he rent the vehicle to drive his wife and dead baby to his village for burial? It was the custom, I knew, and this time I had more than anthropological reasons for facilitating the custom. I felt guilty and I wanted to 'atone' for my guilt, to be 'at one' again with the nurse. I not only agreed that they could use the vehicle, I offered to drive them to the village.

Several hospital staff members rode with us, the nurse sitting in the middle of the back seat with the dead baby on her lap. Most of the way out the car echoed with hymns sung in Swahili. I looked in the rear view mirror: the nurse was singing and tears were streaming down her cheeks.

When we got to her house, we all trooped into the living room and stood or sat, waiting, being with her. The chaplain suggested it was time to pray, and after his prayer of release, each of us who were returning to the hospital walked past her and the baby to say goodbye. When my turn came, she looked me straight in the eye, and said, 'Thank you.'

Thank you? I just killed your baby and you're saying thank you? No, what went on between me and her baby was *my* business – she knew that on some level. As a resident 20 years earlier, I was called to see a cardiology patient as he died. I explained to the family in some detail all that we had tried to do to keep him alive – sharing, apparently, my own debate about the extent of our resuscitation. Later, the cardiologist took me aside and suggested that the place for me to debate my choices was in my closet with God, not with the family. What went on between me and the patient, what choices I'd made in good faith, was *my* business.

However, what was going on with the nurse in Kenya and her baby and me and everyone in that room was God's business, and I had been part of *that* business, and she was thanking me for my part in *that* business. It's not that her cosmology was fatalistic, with death out of human control. Her cosmology was simply big enough to include bad outcomes and mistakes. I was not the end of the line, God was.

Can this view from outside help us take a fresh look at our own healthcare paradigm? Are we aware of its limited scope? Our paradigm gives us plenty of tools to diagnose and to treat, but does it give us an approach to suffering (Chapter 6) and healing (Chapter 10)? Is our scientific, mechanistic paradigm big enough to deal with the bigger questions that are in our patients' minds?

CHAPTER FOUR

Hubris

'He who would be a healer must set great value on seeing truly, hearing truly, understanding truly, and acting truly.' The healer laughed at himself. 'You see why healing can't be a popular vocation? The healer would rather see and hear and understand than have power over men. Most people would rather have power over men than see and hear.'

Ayi Kwei Armah, *The Healers*

All doctors know that Aesculapius is our 'patron saint', but most of us don't know very much about him. His story is interesting and gives us perhaps more insight into our profession than we want.

Aesculapius was the son of Apollo, the Greek god of truth, and Coronis, a beautiful mortal. She, however, spurned Apollo while she was pregnant and he had her killed. By the time of the funeral, however, Apollo felt a pang of grief about his soon-to-be born child, and snatched him away from Coronis as she burned on her funeral pyre. He gave the child Aesculapius to a centaur named Chiron to raise.

Though centaurs, half horse and half man, were generally savage creatures, Chiron was renowned for being good, kind, and wise. He had raised the sons of other notables, but many of those lads were interested only in sport. Aesculapius, however, asked Chiron to teach him about the art of healing. Chiron was pleased to, as he knew much about herbs and incantations. However, Aesculapius surpassed even his wise teacher in his ability to heal and long after his death, people came to his temples and were healed. He is still revered today as the mythical god of medicine and healing.

But that is not the whole story. Because of his great skill and reputation, Aesculapius was given many challenges, among them the request to raise someone from the dead – for a large fee. His patient was Hippolytus, who had died unjustly. It seemed to be a good cause and Aesculapius succeeded in bringing him back to life. But according to Zeus, the chief god and father of Apollo, Aesculapius had gone too far. He, the son of a mortal, had claimed power over death, and that power was reserved only for deity. He had gone beyond human limits in seeking to acquire the attributes of a god. This presumption the Greeks called hubris, and it needed to be punished. Sometimes it was the goddess Nemesis who carried out the punishment but in this case Zeus himself killed Aesculapius with his thunderbolt.

It is interesting that we remember Aesculapius for his healing powers, not for his hubris. Perhaps we don't want to be reminded of the risks in our own profession; perhaps we are content to work in successful Aesculapian temples and forget why Aesculapius himself is no longer there. But there is another story of hubris more familiar to us, that of Prometheus, and it also has links to our profession that we cannot ignore.

The task of creating humanity, according to one Greek legend, was delegated by the gods to Prometheus, whose name means forethought, and his brother Epimetheus, whose name means afterthought. Epimetheus was impulsive and scatterbrained; his brother thoughtful and wise. Epimetheus began first: 'Before making men he gave all the best gifts to the animals, strength and swiftness and courage and shrewd cunning, fur and feathers and wings and shells and the like – until no good was left for men, no protective covering and no quality to make them a match for the beasts. Too late, as always, he was sorry and asked his brother's help. Prometheus, then, took over the task of creation and thought out a way to make mankind superior.' But his solution was not, as I would have thought, to give mankind intelligence or language or opposing thumbs. No, 'he went to heaven, to the sun, where he lit a torch and brought down fire, a protection to men far better than anything else, whether fur or feathers or strength or swiftness.'[1]

For this bold act he earned the reputation among humans as the savior of mankind, but Zeus didn't see it that way. To him, Prometheus had stolen fire from the gods. This was hubris of the first order, acquiring for all people what the gods felt was theirs alone. For punishment, Zeus chained Prometheus to a rock in the Caucasus Mountains and ordered an eagle to come daily and feast on his liver – an eternal punishment since his liver kept regenerating.

Prometheus was eventually freed, we're not sure how. One legend has Hercules killing the eagle and releasing the chains. But for our purposes the more interesting story is one that ties us back to Aesculapius. Zeus's messenger Hermes tells Prometheus:

> *Look for no ending to this agony*
> *Until a god will freely suffer for you,*
> *Will take on him your pain, and in your stead*

Descend to where the sun is turned to darkness,
The black depths of death.

Chiron, the centaur who raised Aesculapius, offered himself and Zeus, in accepting the offer, freed Prometheus.

A common interpretation of this story is that the fire which Prometheus stole from the gods represents technology – including medical technology – and that the more we develop technology, the more we exhibit hubris. A better story to represent the excesses of technology (for those of us disturbed by those excesses) might be that of Pandora (Epimetheus's wife!) when she opened the box and let out all the plagues, sorrows, and mischief the gods had stored in there for mankind. But the Prometheus story is more complex. Did Prometheus save mankind by obtaining for us the essence of technology or open a Pandora's box? Was it redemption or hubris?

Or could it be both? Doesn't medical technology in the hands of humans require great wisdom to know the difference between an aid to healing and hubris? Chiron, the teacher of Aesculapius, had great wisdom and goodness but never hubris; he did not use his skills to control death as Aesculapius did. He perhaps recognized the value of technology for the good of mankind, and was willing to save Prometheus. But he, the wise healer, did not presume to do what only gods could do, and did not presume that there was no cost. He freed Prometheus, but the cost was his own life.

We have, then, three ancient Greek heroes, ready to be mirrors for us of our own profession. There is Aesculapius, known as the healer but punished for his hubris. There is Prometheus, remembered for his hubris yet the bearer of technology that is so crucial to modern medicine. And there is Chiron, the least well known of the three, teacher of the healer, redeemer of the technologist, like the biblical Great Physician in his actions as well as his name, and yet without hubris. When we look into this mirror, what do we see?

As we noted when looking at paradigms, it is difficult to describe our own paradigm. It is even difficult to see ourselves in the mirror of Greek myth. We are trained so thoroughly by our own people in our own paradigm that anything outside it looks strange, antiquated, and – except in reflections like these – irrelevant. We have an 'of course' attitude toward much that we do. Should we scrub our hands and wear sterile gloves before doing surgery? Of course. Should women deliver babies in the hospital? Of course. Should we treat cancer when we find it? Of course. Should we perform CPR on someone whose heart has stopped beating and ventilate someone who has stopped breathing? Of course. These are not questions of opinion or hubris, they are matters relating to our standard of care, and the answers are obvious: Of course.

Once again, however, it is the view from outside which can help us see ourselves better. The Greek myths are outside our time; Africa is outside our place. Let us look at how these outside views will help us see the following.

Consider this story from an Opinion column in the *Guardian Weekly*,[2] reprinted from the *Washington Post*. The writer was commenting on a lawsuit in Virginia in which a lay midwife was charged with manslaughter because the baby of a mother she was attending at home died. Or, it seems, the baby was stillborn, having been breech with a 'compressed' umbilical cord. The situation was clearly 'high risk': the mother was 39 years old having her first baby, her home had no electricity, the baby was breech, and the midwife was 'lay.' The midwife's lawyer argued that she should not be held liable as she was only carrying out the wishes of the parents. The writer of the column agreed: he felt the *parents* should be held liable for manslaughter.

He then entered into a diatribe against people who wanted to do things 'naturally.' 'Natural' childbirth in the last century, he pointed out, naturally led to an infant mortality rate 10 times what it is now. It was a parent's duty, he said, 'to avoid these "natural" phenomena by all possible means' – and we could, with modern medicine.

This case is not very different from the situation with Pamela in Campbell County, Tennessee, about 25 years ago. Pamela had a bone tumor in her thigh and her parents, because of their religion, decided to pray for her healing rather than rely on modern medicine. The Department of Human Services found out and had her removed from the home. She was forced to undergo chemotherapy in Knoxville, since the medical prognosis was that she had no chance of survival without it, but a small chance with it. We don't know what would have happened if the chemotherapy had been started much earlier, but Pamela survived neither prayer nor chemotherapy.

I cannot argue with the medical opinions in either case. I know only too well what happens to infant mortality – and maternal mortality – when most deliveries are done at home; or what happens where chemotherapy is not available. Many African countries have infant mortality rates 10 times that of the USA, and the vast majority of African people with cancer probably die from it. The question is not whether or not modern scientific medicine 'works.' It does.

The question, I think, regards the attitudes of the columnist from the *Washington Post* and of the Tennessee Department of Human Services. In both cases there is the assumption that because medicine can work, we must use it; there is no other way. Both show scorn for people who feel there *are* other ways. In both, acting on a different opinion became legal matters. The problem is not in granting the validity of modern medicine, it is in denying the validity of any other system. That is arrogant; that is presumptuous. That is modern hubris.

Now it may be that this attitude is changing in some segments of Western medicine, especially family medicine. There may be an increasing willingness by doctors to curtail technology at the extremes of life or to accept other approaches to healing. We may be more willing to turn off a respirator on a brain-dead patient or to agree to withhold yet another course of chemotherapy from a patient with metastatic cancer. But the hubris of post-World War II medical advances is still with us – and is sometimes stronger among non-medical people than among health professionals. Our society continues to seek technological solutions to behavioral problems, and continues to ask us to prescribe them.

But it is difficult to see this as presumption, as hubris, when studies can 'prove' the value of the technology. Surely that is not presumption, but simply good sense. Surely everyone agrees that 'pain is normally – indeed, "naturally" – something humans try to avoid,' and that the pain of childbirth is 'today, entirely unnecessary.' To the *Washington Post* writer, that may be obvious but it is not obvious to mothers in America who choose 'natural' unmedicated childbirth, nor is it obvious to most of the people in the 'Two-Thirds World.' Simply because the pain of childbearing can be removed, does that make it 'unnecessary'? How does he know?

It is hard to see the hubris woven through all of our culture until we live in a culture where it is, for the most part, absent. African people are, in general, not arrogant; they defer. They do not force their ways on others; on the contrary, they include other ways with their own. Their thinking is not as exclusive as ours. To them, if a certain way is right, that does not make all other ways wrong. Some of their despotic and obscenely rich presidents are the very antithesis of what Africa is in essence; they are the exceptions that prove the rule.

Now this deferring society lacking hubris can be a two-edged sword. I was talking with an African-American medical student during her first trip to Africa. I was trying to articulate for her some of the wealth that I had gleaned from Africa: the deep family and community ties, the belief in God, the open arms to guests, the ability to forgive (exemplified by Nelson Mandela), the hope – not to mention the music. It was, I said, a seam of gold, buried very deep and not always found, but gold nonetheless – and that I suspected that the black community in America still mined that seam. She sighed; she recognized the truth in what I said and told me that those qualities do not help a community develop or maintain power – and without power, neither American blacks nor Africa can compete in a world where power is increasingly needed even to survive.

She's right, of course. A society that lacks hubris lacks power. Conversely, a power-obsessed society can be so full of hubris that it no longer recognizes it. The very inability to see our hubris is either because we don't have it or because it is so common that we no longer name it.

To get back to the *Washington Post* and the Department of Human Services, both are examples of non-medical institutions that have adopted the hubris of medicine. This is not Prometheus stealing fire or Aesculapius raising the dead, this is the public and legal defense of them. There has been no thunderbolt to wipe out modern Aesculapius; Prometheus is unbound. Where is the Nemesis from the gods? There seems to be none. Possibly hubris is no longer an offense to the gods, but simply common sense. Or possibly there are no gods.

There *seems* to be no Nemesis. But 30 years ago Ivan Illich suggested that not only was the hubris of medicine far advanced, but that its Nemesis was as well. When I read his book *Medical Nemesis: the expropriation of health*[3] shortly after it came out, I vacillated between being offended, on the one hand, and wondering why I was in medicine on the other. When I re-read it 20 years later, I was neither shocked nor threatened. It all seemed obvious.

As Illich sees it, we have followed both Prometheus and Aesculapius. We have used technology to functionally raise the dead and we *are* being 'punished' for this hubris – by the medical system itself. First, he says, is well-known **clinical iatrogenesis**, 'the damage that doctors inflict with the intent of curing' and 'those other torts that result from the doctor's attempt to protect himself against the possibility of a suit for malpractice.'

Beyond this, though, is what he calls **social iatrogenesis**, whereby 'medical practice sponsors sickness by reinforcing a morbid society.' Here, 'medical bureaucracy creates ill-health by increasing stress, by multiplying disability dependence, . . . by lowering the levels of tolerance for discomfort or pain, by reducing the leeway that people are wont to concede to an individual when he suffers, and by abolishing even the right to self-care . . . All suffering is 'hospitalized' and homes become inhospitable to birth, sickness, and death, . . . [and] suffering, mourning, and healing outside the patient role are labeled a form of deviance.'

Finally, Illich sees **cultural iatrogenesis**. Here, 'the so-called health professions have an even deeper, culturally health-denying effect insofar as they destroy the potential of people to deal with their human weakness, vulnerability, and uniqueness in a personal and autonomous way.' This leads to 'the paralysis of healthy responses to suffering, impairment, and death.' 'It sets in when the medical enterprise saps the will of people to suffer their reality.'[4]

In brief, Illich says the Nemesis of our medical hubris is our medical system itself. Aesculapius and Prometheus have become Zeus. They cure our diseases and lengthen our lives, then chain us to the rock of medical technology while their treatments eat away at our ability to take care of ourselves – or even our ability to suffer nobly when nothing can be done.

Despite Illich's devastating critique, in 1975 he remained hopeful. 'The recovery of personal autonomy will,' he wrote, 'be the result of political action reinforcing an ethical awakening. People . . . will limit medical therapies because they want to conserve their opportunity and power to heal.'[5] What has happened since he wrote? Have his predictions of increased autonomy and self-healing come true?

Hardly. We have, however, made some real progress against what he called social iatrogenesis. We no longer hospitalize all suffering – we have hospice, home care, and Do Not Resuscitate orders – and our society has an increased tolerance for 'alternative' forms of treatment. We have made a dent in some of the most obvious forms of medical hubris, and have talked about putting the brakes on some of the most costly forms of runaway technology.

But Illich's hope for a widespread 'recovery of personal autonomy' was a grandiose wish which now sounds naive and dated, a product of the countercultural 'people power' movements that were so vocal when he wrote. Illich himself, in later writings, critiqued and retracted his own optimism.[6] Hopes like these are now being legally crucified in Virginia while the liberal press sits in the gallery cheering. People power is wonderful when it works, but the last 30 years have shown that people power is not likely to radically alter our society's dependence on technology. And our medical system needs technology: Aesculapius and Prometheus work so closely together today that we cannot imagine Aesculapius alone, even though the combination has allowed for an unrestrained hubris which resulted in Medical Nemesis.[7]

Perhaps we need to return to Chiron. To be Chiron, it is not necessary to reject medicine: Chiron taught Aesculapius. Nor is it necessary to reject technology: Chiron redeemed Prometheus. The difference between them, we saw, was that Chiron lacked hubris. Or, to put it positively, he had humility.

Is it possible for a healthcare system to be humble? I don't know; 'humble' is related to the words 'humus' and 'humane', earthy people words, not system or technology words. But doctors are people, and we live on the earth. Illich held out a vague hope that 'the people' would somehow recover the responsibility for their own health. Perhaps a more concrete hope is that doctors will choose to give back to patients the responsibility for their health. It may be that frustration at our patients' impotence and dependence will drive us. But it may also be that the weight of hubris will prove too heavy for some of us, we who really don't want to be gods, and that the way of humility will be the way to freedom.

CHAPTER FIVE

Ethics

[Paul Lacroix said] 'As for us, we conquer a little more of truth each day, thanks to science . . .'
[Diallo thought:] 'They [Europeans] are so fascinated by the returns they get from the implement that they have lost sight of the infinite immensity of the workyard. They do not see that the truth which they discover each day is more and more contracted.'

Cheikh Hamidou Kane, *Ambiguous Adventure*

A short time ago, the following case was heard in a court in Britain, though it could have occurred in America: Siamese twins were born in a hospital in Manchester, England, in August 2000. They were joined at the chest and abdomen, and shared the same heart and lungs. The medical prognosis was that if no surgical procedure was done, they were both likely to die. If surgery was performed, 'Jodie' might live – though with some residual disability likely – and 'Mary' would certainly die, since there was only one heart. At the time of the case, Jodie was more vigorous and Mary had a deformed face and could not cry since the lungs were not in her chest.

The parents came to England for the care of this obviously complicated pregnancy because in their country there was less sophisticated technology. The physicians in Britain offered to surgically separate the twins. The parents, devout Roman Catholics, refused, preferring to 'let nature take its course,' according to the news reports. The hospital took the case to court, which ruled that the surgery should proceed. Lawyers for the parents appealed, and lost.[1] The twins were separated, and Mary died.

The mystery in this case was not the outcome: it doesn't matter. The mystery is deeper: How did it end up in court in the first place? Why was the decision so difficult? And why were the parents' culture – and level of technology they were familiar with – being ignored? The mystery is how medical ethics became so lost.

Legally inappropriate

On the surface, the question of how the case ended up in court is simple: the hospital wanted to do surgery and the parents didn't. They couldn't agree, so they asked the legal system to decide. Apparently there were no other readily available mediators. Apparently the hospital felt strongly enough that they could not simply let the family decide. Apparently the participants saw this not simply as a difference of medical opinion but a question of 'ought,' a moral question – and lacking a commonly agreed moral court, they ended up in a legal court.

The problem, of course, is that courts are set up to decide whether an action is legal or criminal, and only indirectly right or wrong. Consequently, differences of opinion are couched in legal language: 'The judge said that those with parental responsibility could arguably be guilty of the manslaughter of Jodie if they did not act, but guilty of the manslaughter of Mary if they allowed the separation.'[2] To lawyers, this may be an accurate statement of the dilemma. To non-lawyers, it sounds like grandiose language being employed to make a heart-breaking situation melodramatic. Bringing this situation into a court of law makes an already difficult decision impossible.

The problem is not in asking thorny questions, nor in courts doing what they know how to do; the problem is in asking the right question in the wrong place (or the wrong question in the right place). Should a patient with metastatic cancer have to undergo yet another round of toxic chemotherapy? Should a doctor trained by a state-supported medical school be allowed to spend her whole life practicing in Africa – or even in another state? Should an obese diabetic patient with renal failure be considered for a kidney transplant? I can imagine these cases ending up in court, and I can foresee only more dilemmas. These are not fundamentally legal questions, they are ethical questions – and a court of law is the wrong place to settle them.

Ethically confusing

What, then, is wrong with our ethics that we seek legal opinions for ethical questions? Why do we have such difficulty navigating our way through moral questions? Where did our current conception of medical ethics come from?

When I was in medical school in the early 1970s, we did not have a lot of obvious confusion about medical ethics. Most general practitioners, at least, made decisions based on what they thought was best for the patient. We tried to cure and we tried to comfort, because we thought that was best. When it seemed that further attempts at cure were futile, we withheld technology, without being concerned about whether we had 'informed consent' to do so. When we helped people live, and when we 'let' them die, we were basing our decisions on our own inner sense of right and wrong, on culturally determined norms, and on common sense.

It's not that we had no conflicts then. There were already questions about unplugging respirators on brain-dead patients, we did not agree about abortion, and we knew that not everyone who needed healthcare could afford it. We had no easy answers to these dilemmas, but they did not confront us every day. We continued to rely on our own intuition, based on our own values, to decide what was best for our patients.

However, as technology spawned more and more unplug-the-respirator-or-not kind of questions, and as patients realized they were consumers of our services, it became clear that there were questions of value differences that we needed to confront. That opened the way for medical ethicists to reflect on these questions, to help clarify what the issues were.

Medical ethicists did help to clarify, and what became clear was that we physicians were not functioning from an innate universal human ethic, but from our own personal values. They may be good values, but they also may be different from the values of the specialist we were referring to or the values of the patient we were treating. There was no one commonly agreed value system. So when we asked the medical ethicist to help us decide whether or not to pull the plug, we got no direct answer. We needed to consider the values of all the players first, we were told, and then we needed to respect the patient's autonomy.

Because, the medical ethicist reminded us, autonomy has really been the cornerstone of Western society since the Enlightenment. Each of us is a free, responsible individual who should be intimately involved with decisions about his or her healthcare. Perhaps we physicians did not assume this about patients when we used our own values and common sense to decide what to do. Perhaps our whole profession has functioned according to an ethic which is out of date with the rest of Western society. Perhaps we needed to confront the pivotal role and responsibility that our society delegates to the individual.

So, in a postmodern world that cannot agree on 'absolute' values, we needed a set of principles on which to base our ethical reasoning. Autonomy of the individual seemed to give us what we needed: a way to respect our moral diversity. Together with the ancient *non nocere* (do no harm), that gave us two tools we thought would be acceptable for postmodern medical ethics.

Autonomy and *non nocere* are fine tools. The problem, as the case of the Siamese twins so ably demonstrates, is that they cannot always help us to answer our thorny questions, which then get referred to courts of law instead. Let us examine both tools.

'Do no harm' is an excellent foundation. Few if any societies would take issue with this principle. The problem is in using it to decide what to do with the Siamese twins. If we operate, we harm Mary – she dies. If we don't operate, by our inaction we harm both. If we force the parents to accept surgery, we harm their value system. If we agree with them, we harm the hospital's understanding of their mission. We cannot do *no* harm. The principle alone is not enough.

So we come to autonomy. Autonomy doesn't try to tell us what to do, it simply tells us to seek a path consistent with the values of the patient. It asks us to lay aside our own 'oughts' and seek to encourage and strengthen the 'oughts' of the one facing the choice. It is an attempt to help us navigate through thorny ethical questions in a society that does not have a commonly agreed set of moral principles.

The tool may be a good one, but it is difficult to use with children. We cannot respect their autonomously chosen value system before they have developed one, so we try to respect their potential to develop their own value system, even if it is different from their parents'. But even that is difficult. We could recommend that a young child of Jehovah's Witness parents be given a needed blood transfusion since the child may not eventually choose the Jehovah's Witness faith. But giving the blood transfusion does not automatically protect his autonomy: if he chooses the Jehovah's Witness faith later, we have acted against his eventual wishes.

The younger the child, the more the confusion. If we respect the autonomy of very young, even premature children, should we not respect the autonomy of children before they are born? The autonomy argument would seem to argue against abortion, but it then collides with the autonomy of the woman carrying the fetus. Autonomy has not helped us with this, the most common and contentious medical ethical question in America today.[3]

The limits of the autonomy tool are particularly clear with the Siamese twins. If we (medical providers, court) want to defend their autonomy, the case becomes absurd. If we protect Mary's autonomy and potential to choose to live, we cannot operate. If we defend Jodie's, we must operate. Autonomy, the basis of our medical ethics, has failed us.

To review briefly: we in North America and Europe live in a society that has no commonly agreed-upon moral 'absolutes' but we constantly face questions that moral absolutes used to give us direction on. We do not want to impose values on people, so we function according to 'least common denominator' values like 'do no harm,' together with the attempt to respect each person's autonomy and values. These skeleton tools often are not enough to settle our difficult questions, so the questions often end up in court. But legal courts are only intended to decide what is or is not against the law, and often prove inadequate.

The British case of the Siamese twins has exposed the limits of our legal system and of our medical ethics. Hidden within the case, however, may be a clue to an alternative approach to dealing with complex, thorny questions.

Technology is optional

The drama of the Siamese twins was being played out in a British court, but the family involved was not British. They came from a 'remote' community in an unnamed European country, the news reports say, 'which lacked sophisticated medical facilities.' Clearly they carried with them the culture and values of that 'remote' community. Clearly they respected technology enough to go to Britain to deliver their twins, but not so much that they felt they had to partake of whatever technology was offered. Clearly they drew from a set of values other than the 'technological imperative' when they asked that their twins not be operated on and nature be left to take its course. They had a view from outside.

However, they could have been a British couple who did not want to force Mary to die so that Jodie could live. Or a British couple who did not want technology to be the foundation of their ethics. For in fact, it's the technological ability to separate these twins which precipitated this ethical and legal dilemma. In the parents' home community, there would be no ethical dilemma, no accusations of manslaughter, no legal case. Nature would take its course, and the twins would likely die. That was the parents' wish.

But (the response is obvious) we *do* have technology in the West. We do have the ability to save and prolong life. We have a standard of medical care which we all agree on, and failure to follow this standard is unethical or even illegal. The standard is there to promote life and health. Who could disagree?

Plenty of people. Christian Scientists, Jehovah's Witnesses, and other denominations that believe in miraculous healing disagree. Countless people who follow alternative healing systems (homeopathy, naturopathy, etc.) disagree. The Amish disagree. Some Native Americans disagree. And clearly the parents of the Siamese twins disagreed. Our standard based on technology is not as widely accepted as it seems.

What then is the role of technology? I propose that technology is *always* optional, that it never need be the foundation for ethical decisions. Our ability to perform extraordinary technological procedures should never be an imperative. When there is a dispute between parties about the use of a certain technology, the ethical question can be approached this way: assume the technology does not exist, answer the ethical question based on the motives and desires of all the parties, *then* offer the technology. It is always optional. Technology cannot alter our moral foundations. Two-thirds or more of the world's people do not have access to the kind of technology that precipitates this ethical confusion, yet they still can function very morally and ethically.

To see how this approach might work in practice, let us return to the Siamese twins in Britain. The parents have been offered surgery, realize both twins will likely die without it, and one undoubtedly will with it. They choose against surgery. The hospital disagrees, wanting to save the life of at least one. If we consider how the case would look if there were no technology, the twins would likely die – and letting them die would obviously not be manslaughter. It would not be a legal case at all.

But since surgery does exist, it is important to ask why the parents are deciding against it. Do they, for example, have a history of child abuse or neglect, and could they be refusing surgery because they didn't want these offspring in the first place? Is their refusal of surgery an indirect way to get rid of some children they would otherwise actually kill? Or are they normal caring parents, troubled by the thought that a technological response would definitely eliminate the life of Mary, and likely make Jodie dependent on further technology for some time?

It is equally important to ask why the hospital is so committed to having the surgery done. Do they have economic motives and are afraid of losing the business? Are they concerned that a precedent may be set if surgery is refused, and the status of the technological medicine may suffer? Or do they truly believe that their procedure is in the best interests of the family?

It is clear that seeing technology as optional does not eliminate ethical questions. We still need to consider why one party might be so adamant about using a certain technology and the other so adamant against. In fact, it may be that seeing technology as optional helps us to clarify the more important underlying ethical questions. The deeper questions are not about *whether* to use technology, but *why*.

Focusing on technology uncovers an ethical problem of another order altogether. The concentration of technology in the One-Third World is itself an ethical dilemma. That judges in Britain spend time agonizing over the possible manslaughter of one Siamese twin or the other while Third-World children die of readily treatable and preventable infections is itself an ethical scandal. If technology has truly become part of the moral foundation of the West, then it would be unethical to pull it away and distribute it world-wide – and equally unethical to condemn the rest of the world to poor health and death in its absence. We're back to the judge proclaiming that no matter what we do, we have killed someone.

But if life-saving technology is always only an option, then we are free to re-examine it, to consider where there is an excess, to imagine how the resources spent on it could be redeployed for low-level life-saving technology elsewhere. Realizing that technology is optional frees us from worshiping it, and frees us to use it intelligently.

SUFFERING

CHAPTER SIX

Suffering

... In [Senegal] man is closer to death. He lives on more familiar terms with it ... There existed between death and myself an intimacy made up at the same time of my terror and my expectation. Whereas here [France] death has become a stranger to me. Everything combats it, drives it back from men's bodies and minds ...

Cheikh Hamidou Kane, *Ambiguous Adventure*

Wednesday morning, January 8, 1997. National Public Radio news. The Supreme Court is about to hear testimony on physician-assisted suicide for terminally ill patients. And new studies are coming out adding to the debate on whether or not there is a Gulf War syndrome. In the first story, the question is what we do about the suffering of the terminally ill; in the second, it is what we do about the suffering of war veterans. In both there is an unspoken cry of the need to relieve human suffering.

We don't understand suffering.

I

I began to learn about suffering from Chief's funeral in Tanzania. I remember clearly when he died. We all knew him: he had worked in several departments of the hospital, knew more about leprosy than most of us ever would, and continued to serve where he was needed. But his death was memorable not just because he was well known; it was memorable because it was sudden. It seemed that children were always dying suddenly, from causes we could never determine. But unlike in America, African adults don't have much cardiovascular disease, and sudden death from myocardial infarction, arrhythmias or even pulmonary emboli is uncommon. But Chief probably did have an MI or a pulmonary embolism. He collapsed, gurgled, and died.

I was in another village when he died, but I heard about it later. There were shrieks, and more shrieks, as the news spread through our village of Shirati. Chief was an institution not just at the hospital, but also in the village. He died at home in his own village, so many people who knew him were around to mourn and wail – and his tribe really mourned and wailed.

But that was just the beginning. His adult children had gotten further education and moved to bigger cities for jobs. They had to be notified; they had to come home for the funeral. For several days they gathered at the homestead in Shirati, eating together and hosting the large number of mourners who came daily to pay respects. In the middle of the fortnight of feasting and socializing was the several hour long funeral and burial. It was at the burial that I saw what suffering was.

After the sermons and the prayers, several people carried the home-made casket from the church to Chief's homestead. I remember the mid-day heat; I remember wanting to find some shade as we stood around the freshly dug grave and the young men lowered the casket into the hole. I was standing near one of Chief's daughters as the casket was being lowered and I remember her almost uncontrollable crying and shrieking. She was suffering.

Then at the final prayer, as they were getting ready to shovel the dirt back in, she elbowed her way forward to see the casket in the hole. I couldn't see but I could hear the sound I always listen for, the final sound of dirt rattling on the coffin lid. She was apparently looking for that same final goodbye because just after I heard it, I saw her coming back from the hole, drying her eyes, and I heard her say, 'There!' It was finished.

Chief's daughter was suffering and the one thing I would not want to do as a physician would be to take away that suffering. She was feeling all the pain of her father's premature, unexpected death and she was suffering in the ways her culture had taught her to suffer. Built in to that suffering was a way to express her pain out loud; built in also was a way to physically get 'closure,' to let go, knowing that her father was in the earth and would not come back.

We, of course, have similar culturally determined funeral rites that help us deal with the pain of death. But I sense that we still have trouble making sense out of death, especially when it is premature. On the way back from another funeral in Tanzania, an American friend was comparing the unexpected death of his brother-in-law, who was in his 40s, with the unexpected death of the pastor whose funeral we had just attended. He said that at the American funeral of his brother-in-law, many people commented on the tragedy of him being cut off in his prime, implying that his life was incomplete when he died. The death was, in other words, senseless.

At the African funeral we had just been to, on the other hand, the eulogies assumed that the pastor had completed the cycle of life allotted him. It was no less painful for the people to come to grips with *his* premature death but they had a world-view which helped them to know what to do with this pain, which helped them to suffer, to make sense out of the pain.

There is a difference between pain and suffering. Pain is noxious feelings; suffering is the experience, determined by culture, of bearing those feelings.[1] The Latin origin of these words makes this clear: **pain** comes from *poena*, meaning penalty or punishment; **suffer** comes from *sufferre*, from *sub* = under + *ferre* = to bear.

When I eat too much, I feel pain in my stomach, the penalty for dietary excess. When I smash my fist into a brick wall, I feel pain in my knuckles, the punishment for handling my anger in such a stupid way. When someone else smashes his fist into my face, the pain I feel may be punishment for something stupid I said but I may also be an innocent victim. When I feel the chronic pain of breast or prostate cancer metastasized to my bones, I may wonder if I'm being punished for something. Or I may be angry and depressed because I know I did nothing to deserve such punishing pain.

Regardless of the cause, my duty as a physician calls for me to help relieve and prevent pain, whether it is punishment or consequence or simply a warning sign. I also will likely want to help relieve suffering, especially if I view suffering according to the way it is popularly understood, which is something like 'chronic bad pain.' If *that* is the suffering I want to help relieve, I will be doing no damage to my patients or their coping mechanisms by helping eliminate it. If suffering has already been reduced to simply the experience of 'chronic bad pain,' only cruelty would want to preserve that.

But chronic bad pain is not the same as suffering. At least it didn't used to be and still isn't in most of the world. *Suffering* is how we *bear under* pain, in the same way that *transferring* is *bearing* or carrying something *over*, and *conferring* is *bearing* or discussing a matter *together*. Suffering is the culturally determined ways in which we bear our pain, the ways in which Chief's daughter came to grips with her father's death. 'Culture makes pain tolerable by integrating it into a meaningful setting; . . . by interpreting its necessity . . .'[2] Suffering is to pain as inflammation is to infection. Both suffering and inflammation hurt and as physicians, we want to help relieve the hurt. But our main task must be to address the underlying pain and infection.

But what is our response when we can do nothing about the underlying pain? Traditionally we have talked of 'palliative measures,' of using whatever technology we have to decrease the pain we cannot eliminate. And because of our desire to reduce pain, we have not thought about *helping* our patients suffer, we have instead sought ways to eliminate the suffering. Our focus is on getting rid of pain, not giving it meaning – because for many of us in our culture, chronic and unremitting or terminal pain has no meaning.

It is not a very big step from admitting that chronic pain has no meaning to seeking legal sanction for physician-assisted suicide. If significant numbers of people in our culture agree that chronic or terminal pain is unnecessary – if they cannot bear under the pain, cannot suffer – and if the job of physicians is to eliminate pain, then why shouldn't we help them get rid of pain permanently? For those that can't bear it, don't we have an obligation to help them end their lives if they request it?

There are two 'ifs' in the last paragraph which lead to the inevitability of physician-assisted suicide. Each needs closer attention.

'If they cannot bear under the pain, cannot suffer . . .' Many people cannot. '[T]he term "suffering" has become almost useless for designating a realistic response because it evokes superstition, sadomasochism, or the rich man's condescension to the lot of the poor . . . [T]he ability of individuals to face their reality, to express their own values, and to accept inevitable and often irremediable pain and impairment, decline, and death' has been undermined.[3]

Ivan Illich blames 'the medical enterprise' and 'professionally organized medicine' for this undermining of the individual's ability to cope with irremediable pain and death. His arguments about our role are indeed compelling. The focus of our biomedical paradigm is on the mechanisms of pain and the techniques of its relief, and it has been remarkably successful. It works so well that we have stopped trying to live with pain, waiting only for the next technology that will take it away.[4]

It's not that pain is inherently intolerable, though; culturally determined suffering can help us to bear it. But some people have lost their cultural and religious roots and are truly unable to suffer. The question of physician-assisted suicide is simply a sad admission of this loss.

'If the job of physicians is to eliminate pain . . .' Of course our job is to reduce pain, but the important question here concerns the 'bottom line' of our profession, for *which* bottom line we hold to will have great significance for how we view physician-assisted suicide. One bottom line we are familiar with is to preserve life, and people holding this view form the core of the opposition to physician-assisted suicide. It doesn't matter how insufferable the pain is, they say; we cannot preserve life by helping to end it.

It's an honorable position but it has a problem. When 'preserve life' becomes 'preserve life at all cost', and this commitment is aided by technology which can maintain biological life (brain waves, respiration, heart beats) almost indefinitely, we have gone from common sense to nonsense, from compassion to hubris. The 'quality of life' critiques have been a valuable balance to this bottom line, but have not abolished it. Many of us still put terminally ill people on respirators; we still spend far too many of our healthcare dollars on the last few weeks of life.

Well then, if 'preserve life' isn't our bottom line, then perhaps 'eliminate pain' (or 'remove suffering' in its contemporary meaning) is our ultimate responsibility. It also is an honorable goal but it too has a problem. In a culture that is losing its ability to suffer and can no longer tell the difference between pain and suffering, our obsessive commitment to eliminating pain may only make the pains we can't relieve more intolerable. We are then obligated to consider the next step, which is helping someone permanently end their pain. This is not the hubris of controlling life, it's the hubris of scheduling death.

Yet there is a third bottom line, also old and honorable, which may help us navigate between these two extremes of hubris. Before technology could preserve life, but also before we had lost our ability to suffer, physicians saw their bottom line as being with patients in their suffering. After performing the surgery or administering the medicine of the day, often with limited hopes of success, compassionate physicians did not abandon their patients; they were with them in their suffering. The word *compassion*, in fact, means exactly that: suffering with.

Has the advent of effective medicines and surgeries changed this bottom line? In a culture that is losing its ability to suffer, isn't it even more important that physicians, especially family physicians, walk with their patients as they face this daunting technology? And in those situations where the technology cannot eliminate the pain, isn't the compassionate response still to be with our patients as they try to make sense out of it?

Perhaps the critical question is not the one facing the Supreme Court. The question of physician-assisted suicide is an admission that we are losing our ability to suffer. But we should not get side-tracked into thinking that a legal verdict solves the problem. The best a legal verdict will do for us is to produce a stand-off much like the ongoing abortion question. No matter what the current legal status of abortion is, there will be a committed group seeking to change it – and diverting attention from the deeper questions of sexual union and procreation. Concentrating on abortion – or physician-assisted suicide – is like trying to close the barn door after the cows are out. We do need to decide whether the door should be open or closed but let us not forget that, regardless of the laws, our patients are hurting, are trying to suffer, and the compassionate bottom line is to simply be with them.

II

If the debate on physician-assisted suicide highlights our inability to comprehend suffering, the argument over the Gulf War syndrome points to one reason why: our ignorance of consequences.

One day in Tanzania, I was brimming with pride about my latest description of development. Development work was what we were all supposed to be doing, helping people move ahead socially and economically. But sometimes it seemed to me that it was an impossible task, so I had decided that 'development is swimming upstream.' My thinking was this: I always felt like I was going against some current when I tried to help people release their own potential. It seemed like the cards were stacked against that process. It took such effort, and we made such little progress. Yet we had duped ourselves into thinking that if enough of us swam upstream, we could change the direction of flow of the river. The whole idea seemed absurd.

I presented this image to Magiri, a friend visiting from another village. He was trained to the level of physician's assistant, now working in a program of primary healthcare development.

'Do you understand what I mean?' I asked.

'Not exactly,' he said.

So I tried in Swahili, using my hands to demonstrate: 'There is a river running this way; perhaps it's the economy of a country. Some people aren't benefiting from that economy, so we say they need development. But development efforts often go against the flow of the economy. We jump in and swim upstream. Sometimes we are on a raft and we paddle furiously against the current. Big development projects even have engines on their boats, and they go way upstream – as long as they have fuel. Then we ask local people to join us in struggling against the current. Should we be surprised when so few of them join us – except on the big boats? Isn't it ludicrous to imagine we can make the river go the other way just because we are?'

Magiri answered in English. 'If you have read anything about aquatic life . . .' he began, and I leaned forward wide-eyed, wondering what was coming next. He looked like he was preparing for a lengthy, convoluted response: '. . . you know that with aquatic animals, anything floating downstream is dead.' That was it.

My metaphor melted. My assumption was that we development workers were the only ones struggling upstream and I, the prophet among us, was treading water, shaking the wet hair out of my eyes, and saying, 'Wait a minute! This is crazy!' But Magiri was saying, no, we have all been struggling for our survival long before you came. He was saying that struggling against odds, or suffering, is a characteristic not of development but of life. He was taking my metaphor a step farther than I had and telling me that I could either struggle upstream, or float down, dead.

Magiri knew – as all people in poor countries know, and as poor people in our country know on a different level – that life is never handed to us on a silver platter. There is a struggle simply to live, and some consequences of that struggle are that we get tired and confused and frustrated. And hurt. Magiri knew that, and knew that our choices were to give up and die, or to continue struggling to live, and to bear the consequences of that struggle. To *bear under* the pain of that struggle: to suffer.

What our culture doesn't seem to understand is that suffering is a part of life, a 'natural' part of life, not an aberration that always needs to be eliminated. The debate about the Gulf War 'syndrome' illustrates this. Interviews with veterans of the first Gulf War have apparently shown that they have significantly more physical symptoms (such as headache, joint pains, memory lapses) than people in the armed services who did not go to the Gulf. This has led to a search for a toxin used against them – a chemical or biological weapon – but none has been proven. A footnote to the National Public Radio news story was that veterans of all wars have more physical symptoms than recruits who do not fight.

It is of course appropriate to look for toxic agents, either agents used against allied soldiers or by them, or even an unexpected consequence of prophylactic measures used to try to protect them. It may prove useful to name the cause of their suffering. But we should not restrict our search to physical causes only. There are emotional and spiritual consequences to waging a war that kills 100 000 people from the other side, even if only 100 of our own died. It should be no surprise that our veterans are suffering after such an experience.

And we should be very cautious about trying to 'eliminate' their suffering or 'compensate' them for it. What our society needs is a way to *help* them suffer, to even join them in their suffering. As we corporately lose the ability to make sense out of pain, ours or our 'enemy's', we leave our soldiers with appalling amounts of unprocessed emotional pain. Any war is a holocaust but what happens to soldiers in contemporary wars, soldiers whose culture has never taught them how to suffer? We are aware of the epidemic of post-traumatic stress syndrome following Vietnam. What happened to the soldiers who fought in Korea? In World War II? What did they do with their pain?

We didn't think about this right after World War II. We won and we wanted to get on with our lives – and we did. But what happened to the pain, the suffering, originating in that holocaust? Our elderly patients are the soldiers of that war. Are they carrying some of the pain, still unprocessed? Are their children and grandchildren?

Are we?

The disintegration of the American nuclear family followed closely on the heels of the broad-based social challenges of the 1960s. But the young people who were at the center of that important and sometimes chaotic decade were the children of World War II veterans. They – we – grew up in homes where no one talked about that war, where no one suffered and mourned openly about that fracture through the middle of the 20th century. Our parents, many of whom also lived through the Great Depression, set about rebuilding after World War II. They worked, and never finished suffering. The hidden family violence of the 1950s and 1960s which was a mirror of that war became the open family violence of the 1970s and beyond. The irony of the US dollar getting stronger on world markets, while the US family weakens, is too obvious to overlook.

Again, it seems that we are dealing with matters beyond the scope of medicine. We can effectively manipulate many disease processes but where we cannot cure, we are only technicians of pain for a people who have forgotten how to suffer. We continue to make great strides in manipulating disease but little progress in managing suffering. No surprise, really: caring for people who cannot suffer is like treating infections in people who have lost their immune systems. We have an epidemic of AIDS of the soul.

We have made some progress with AIDS, but the best we can hope for in the near future is managing a chronic disease, not eliminating a curable one. In the process, physicians who work with AIDS patients have emphasized the need to be with patients.[5] Should we offer anything less to all of our patients?

CHAPTER SEVEN

Chronic disease – 1

'What did Damfo [the healer] actually do to you?' 'He didn't do things to me,' replied Jesiwa. 'He never pushed me. The opposite was the way he treated me. Sometimes I was in a hurry to do something. He would urge me to hold back a bit and think of the thing I wanted to do, to make sure that was really what I needed to do. He never pushed me. And he never deceived me.'

Ayi Kwei Armah, *The Healers*

There was a woman who had a flow of blood for twelve years, and who had suffered much under many physicians, and had spent all that she had, and was no better but rather grew worse.

Mark 5:25–6

I'm fascinated by how doctors disagree (often by sneering) and even more fascinated by what they disagree about. The big disagreements are less about scientifically proven facts than about general approaches or emphases. Surgeons, whose surgeries often 'cure' people, pity internists because the internists can't seem to get rid of the diseases they treat. Public health people boast because their vaccines prevent disease, and at a fraction of the cost of treating it. Specialists quietly demonstrate their superiority to generalists by ordering extensive and esoteric tests. These back-door disagreements are usually based on something true but some of us get so enthusiastic about the small piece of truth we are entrusted with that we use it as a weapon instead of a tool. Yet we still think of ourselves as healers.

The care of chronic diseases, from whatever cause, provides an excellent opportunity for this kind of disagreement. Chronic diseases cause such suffering that any progress – a preventive vaccine, a surgical or medical cure, a symptom-relieving or life-enhancing modality – is welcome; and those who deliver the new treatment sometimes just can't help boasting and sneering. We even see this attitude in the Bible. Luke, the physician, when telling the story of the woman who had been bleeding chronically, reveals only that none of his compatriots had been able to heal her. It was the lay writer Mark who gave us the extended description quoted above. And when Luke records the healing, he has Jesus say only 'Go in peace' but Mark tells us that Jesus said 'Go in peace *and be freed from your suffering.*' This wasn't Jesus sneering, it was Mark exposing a troubling failure of Luke's profession.

We have clearly not conquered all these failures in the treatment of chronic disease. In fact, by preventing death in some acute diseases, we have 'created' many new chronic diseases. Let us, then, look at some stages that we, in North America at least, have gone through in our approach to chronic diseases.

At the beginning of the 20th century, around the time of William Osler, physicians were adept at diagnosing many common chronic conditions by their clinical signs. They could recognize heart failure, diabetes, gout, epilepsy, strokes, psychosis, many cancers, and a host of other chronic diseases, but could do little to treat any of them. Their role was confined to diagnosis, prognosis, and palliation.

By the middle of the 20th century, medicine was developing treatment modalities for almost everything: some were drugs that could 'cure' chronic diseases (such as medicines for tuberculosis) but most were drugs that provided relief without actually 'curing' the disease; many did not even slow the progression of the disease. People with heart failure, schizophrenia, and epilepsy all felt better, and some were even free of their symptoms, but their underlying disease pathology remained unchanged.

The end of the 20th century brought us yet another paradigm in our approach to chronic disease. We are no longer comfortable 'merely' relieving symptoms. Now we can change the course of some diseases, especially diabetes, hypertension, and heart failure, by protecting the 'end-organs' that are usually damaged by those diseases over time. We can also diagnose earlier the diseases that commonly accompany aging – hardening of the arteries (atherosclerosis) and softening of the bones (osteoporosis) – and give drugs to attenuate their development. In addition, we have new techniques to detect very early and treatable stages of cancer – pap smears, mammography, and colonoscopy. Though not all of these techniques and drugs are recent, the paradigm of aggressive management of all people who have *or might get* a chronic disease is new.

There are some diseases, of course, which do not keep pace with this historical pattern. For example, with some strokes we are still in the Osler stage. On the other hand, by the time family medicine was born (1969), we were already talking about protecting end-organs in diabetes and hypertension, and we had long since begun cancer screening. The overall paradigm in the middle of the 20th century still followed Jesus' dictum: 'It is not the healthy who need a doctor, but the sick.' By the end of the century, however, Western physicians and their patients came to believe that all people need doctors – not only to manage the diseases they already have without knowing it but also to prevent *by taking medications* diseases for which they are at risk.

Every new medical paradigm challenges both doctors and their patients. Look, for example, at the move from clinical diagnosis with marginally effective treatment to laboratory diagnosis and medicines to improve or eliminate symptoms. Doctors who had previously used their hands, eyes, and ears to diagnose, and their presence to comfort, now needed to interpret highly technical laboratory tests and prescribe long-term multi-drug therapies. Patients, too, needed to change their understanding of disease. In Osler's time, chronic disease was either progressive (diabetes, heart failure), leading to death, or stable (paralysis, blindness), requiring no ongoing treatment. Now there was a new category: chronic disease whose progression was to be prevented by *the patient* taking medicine every day.

Doctors changed, and so did patients. It was a good change, mostly, because patients were living longer and feeling better. There were, however, some trade-offs. Because doctors were spending more time interpreting lab tests and calculating drug dosages, they had less time to comfort. We never consciously abandoned this role; it simply became optional. Patients too began to evolve. As chronic disease became more and more the responsibility of the doctor, patients became more dependent on doctors, not only for the treatment of their disease but also for support in living with their disease. Patients were more active in management than formerly – *they*, after all, had to take their own medicine – but it was medicine prescribed by and available only through the doctor. Their improved prospects for health and happiness bound them ever closer to the medical profession.

These evolutions in the roles of doctors and patients prepared both for the paradigm shift at the end of the 20th century. Doctors had become adept technicians, able to fine-tune the medication regimens for the increasing number of people who were chronic patients – now including those who were being identified as patients because they had an abnormal lab finding or disease risk. And patients had learned that they needed doctors (in much the same way that they 'needed' electricity) and were more or less ready to *be* patients and to take treatments that were ordered.

Now the foregoing description may be accurate for those who can afford 'state of the art' medical care in North America, and who have stable enough lives to make medicine taking a priority. However, the Third World has not yet joined this latest paradigm shift, nor have many in America's 'third world' communities. In many parts of Africa, for many diseases, we are still at the Osler stage. For example, we can diagnose AIDS clinically but in many places we can offer very little to change the course of the disease, though this is changing rapidly. Even where we can function according to the mid-20th century paradigm, offering insulin for diabetes or effective medicines for heart failure or AIDS, many people can't afford these long-term medicines. And while doctors may have shifted their paradigm of treatment, many patients haven't. The concept of taking medicines for the rest of one's life is still quite literally foreign. Doctors who work in America's poor communities often find the same gap between how they view treatment and how their patients view it.

If there is thus some difficulty for doctors and their patients even in shifting out of the Osler paradigm for chronic disease care, what then is the role of the new paradigm for the Third Worlds? This question is particularly pertinent for Westerners involved in medical education in the Third World, as well as practitioners among America's poor, both of whom are sometimes accused of practicing a 'lower' standard of care.

To put the question more boldly: Is there a role for expensive 'preventive' drugs in places where patients do not yet take 'standard' drugs? Do we really *want* to offer all of them the 'privilege' of becoming patients? Are we satisfied, even in the West, with the increasing dependency on medications, which is the 'side effect' of the new paradigm?

Let us return to the biblical woman with the hemorrhage. She was frustrated, not only by her chronic disease but also by the medical profession. In her case the doctors hadn't helped her – but are patients today who are bound to the medical profession with their chronic diseases any less trapped because they get some relief from symptoms or protection of their end-organs? The effect of Jesus' miracle was not only to release the woman from her chronic disease but also to release her from the medical system. The same was true for the lame fellow who stayed for 38 years by the Pool of Bethesda: he was immobilized not only by his disease but also by his 'maybe next time' hope to be healed in the water. He was so captivated by that system that he didn't even ask Jesus for healing; Jesus approached him and asked if he wanted to get well. Under the new end-of-century paradigm, however, neither of these chronic disease patients would be free from the medical system after their miracle. The woman would be offered hormones at menopause (at least in the 1990s), mammography, and drugs to prevent osteoporosis. The man would need his blood pressure and lipids monitored, and his colon endoscoped.

Now it's obvious that if a medical system can afford to make everyone in society patients, *and* the people in that society readily accept this role, the criticism that they are 'trapped' by the medical system is empty. But not everyone can afford to be on chronic medications, not everyone can remember to take medicines every day, and not everyone *wants* to be a patient. Especially in poor areas of the US and in Third World countries, people have far more pressing priorities than whether or not they might have a hip fracture at age 78 or whether or not their kidneys will be damaged by their diabetes when they can't even afford insulin.

What then should practitioners and educators in Third World communities do with this latest paradigm of chronic disease management? We cannot ignore this new mandate, nor can we assume that there are no benefits in screening and preventive drugs. On the other hand, it is a charade to prescribe according to it when our patients cannot or will not comply. We need to ask at least two questions, informed by a view from outside, that may help us clarify how much of this new paradigm to practice and teach.

First, we need to look at *how much* the new preventive drugs improve outcome, not just whether or not the improvements are statistically significant. For example, in severely ill diabetic patients, insulin makes a difference between living for only three days and living for three more years – or 13 or 30. Will the newer preventive and protective medicines add years to diabetic patients' lives, or only months?

There are similar questions about screening. Screening mammography reportedly reduces mortality from breast cancer in women over 50 by 20–30%. That means that in a given population, if 100 women usually die from breast cancer, screening that population with mammography would mean only 70–80 women die. That's good for the 20–30 women whose lives are saved but four out of five women still die from the disease even when screened for it. Compare this to an African village that usually loses 100 children to measles. If every child in that village is vaccinated, likely no one will die from measles. We who teach and work in Third World communities need to choose which statistically significant results are significant enough to introduce in communities that can barely afford, or have trouble utilizing, even the standard treatments.

There is an important corollary to this first question: Have the studies which prove the effects of the new drugs and screening tests been done in Third World communities? If not, then how applicable are the resulting recommendations for those communities? Possibly the recommendations do apply throughout America, but what about in Africa where the disease patterns are entirely different?

Second, we need to openly confront the dependence on the medical system that these new drugs and screening tests produce. We who work in under-served communities often talk about 'empowerment.' Do we empower a young woman to avoid cervical cancer more when she accepts the habit of regular pap smears or when she accepts healthier sexual habits? Have we empowered a patient with a high cholesterol more by obtaining adherence to a medication regimen or by obtaining adherence to a sensible diet? The immediate response is that our efforts should not be 'either/or.' True – but which activity is more *empowering*? As physicians, our expertise is on the technical side more than the behavioral side, and we offer what we've got. If we are really interested in empowering our patients, we should consider the effect of making them more dependent on us.

These are thorny, contentious questions, even for the non-poor in North America. Chronic disease causes such anguish for everyone that when a surgeon really produces a cure or a researcher develops an effective vaccine, we can understand the boasting. But most chronic diseases still plague us and are even more chronic than they used to be as we live longer with them.

However, for those of us who work or teach in Third World communities, the questions aren't that difficult and the answers are equally clear. We rarely need to agonize over what to offer our patients because they, and often the system serving them, cannot afford the new paradigm. For these people, health is a gift like the sun, not a utility like electricity. When they are healthy, they confront the struggles of life; when health fails, they seek us.

Maybe that's the way it ought to be.

CHAPTER EIGHT

Chronic disease – 2

I do not contest the quality of the truth which science discloses. But it is a partial truth . . .

Cheikh Hamidou Kane, *Ambiguous Adventure*

I recently attended a one-day continuing medical education seminar on diabetes and the newly named 'metabolic syndrome' among Native Americans. The new name came about because of the recognition that diabetes was often accompanied by several other conditions such as high blood pressure and high cholesterol. Despite the acknowledgment that diet and exercise were important in treatment of this syndrome, there was general agreement that most patients would need to take many different drugs, as many as 5–10, to adequately control all the symptoms. During the last question session, I commented on a recent academic article entitled 'Clinical Inertia'[1] which suggested that the failure to adequately control the parts of the metabolic syndrome was due to doctors' failure to be aggressive enough. I asked if there wasn't also social or cultural or patient inertia contributing to poor control. The speaker's response was that patient inertia was 'ubiquitous' but that evidence showed that counseling (for diet, exercise, and appropriate taking of medicines) was effective – in one out of 20 people. The next question was about the pharmacological control of serum lipids.

The question of diabetes control is important. Between one-third and two-thirds of Native Americans have diabetes, depending on the tribe. Probably one in four Americans overall have diabetes, and two-thirds of American adults are overweight and thus potentially 'pre-diabetic.' All of these percentages have increased greatly in the last generation or two. Clearly diabetes and the metabolic syndrome are an American epidemic.

As with any epidemic, American medicine has responded with research, excellent research, and plenty of it. The research confirms that the combination of inactivity, obesity, and a high-fat diet brings on diabetes and the metabolic syndrome, especially in people with a genetic tendency, such as Native Americans. Research also shows that exercise and diet are helpful in controlling the syndrome, but that few people achieve adequate control without medications. Now since this is a syndrome with many parts (high blood sugar, high blood lipids, high blood pressure, high body weight), each part has its own set of medicines; hence the 5–10 medicines that most people will have prescribed for them. And these medicines are not just prescribed for theoretical reasons: each one has been shown by research to improve a part of the syndrome, and better control of the syndrome decreases morbidity and mortality.

The question of whether or not patients actually take all of those medicines seems to be of less interest to the researchers. The expert who answered my question seemed to assume that often patients did *not* take all their medications – patient inertia, he said, was ubiquitous – and then told me what evidence showed I could do effectively for only 5% of those people. We have, then, an epidemic disease, brought on by an undisciplined 'lifestyle,' being treated with numerous discipline-requiring medications. The treatment requires precisely what is lacking in the first place yet research continues apace for new drugs.

In 1959 Rene Dubos wrote this:

> As was the case for the great epidemics, two kinds of medical philosophy are guiding the approach to the control of these modern epidemics. One is the search for drugs capable of reaching the site of the disease within the body of the patient. The other is the attempt to identify those aspects of modern life thought to be responsible for the disease problems peculiar to our times . . . While the search for the magic bullets continues, other studies are revealing that the environment in which the individual lives and his manner of living are of great importance in determining his susceptibility to the diseases of modern times . . . The sickness of the individual is not readily differentiated from the sickness of society.[2]

In 1983, Stephen Kunitz referred to the same two kinds of medical philosophy in his discussion of disease among Navajo people over the last century. He concluded:

> Since many of the most serious and difficult [contemporary] problems . . . appear to be rooted in traditional patterns of ecological adaptation and social organization, they are likely to be especially refractory to medical intervention and will respond only to profound changes in Navajo life. To the degree that the health professions deal with these issues, they will move more and more into ambiguous regions where medical expertise may often be misapplied and even wrong in respect of the explanations it offers and treatments it recommends.[3]

While it is clear that both kinds of Dubos's 'medical philosophy' are guiding the current approach to the control of the metabolic syndrome, my impression is that the search for magic bullets is upstaging the attempts to treat the sickness of society. Perhaps the medical researchers would contend that it's their job to look for the magic bullets, and someone else's job to find ways to ensure that the patients are taking those magic bullets, and someone else's still to address the sickness of society. Perhaps the society would prefer magic bullets, even with the risk that 'medical expertise may be misapplied or even wrong.' Perhaps the existence of health education and public health programs frees the medical researchers – and many doctors and patients – to think only of magic bullets. No one rejects public health; it simply plays second fiddle to clinical medicine. And more often than not, the two fiddles are not playing in harmony; they are simply playing different songs.

We need a view from outside and again, Africa provides that view. Thabo Mbeki, President of South Africa, was criticized – or rather crucified – in the news media at the beginning of his presidency because of his stance on HIV/AIDS and antiretroviral drug therapy. The media accused him of not believing that HIV causes AIDS, of ignoring the AIDS epidemic in his country, and even of precipitating the death of people by denying them medicines. Possibly one reason why the news media were unable to understand Mbeki's approach to HIV is the dominance of clinical medicine's hope-for-magic-bullets that characterizes our approach to diabetes. Yet few if any of the news articles I had read quoted what Mbeki actually said. So I looked. The following are quotes from Mbeki speeches and interviews:

May 6, 2000 'What we knew was that there is a virus, HIV. The virus causes AIDS.' '[In 1985, predominant transmission of AIDS was among male homosexuals in both South Africa and the US and Western Europe.] The situation has not changed in the United States up to today, nor in Western Europe with regard to homosexual transmission. But here it changed very radically in a short period of time and increased very radically in a short period of time. Why?'[4]

July 9, 2000: '. . . [E]xtreme poverty is the world's biggest killer and the greatest cause of ill health and suffering across the globe . . . [O]ne of the consequences of this crisis is the deeply disturbing phenomenon of the collapse of immune systems among millions of our people, such that their bodies have no natural defense against attack by many viruses and bacteria . . . [I]t seemed to me that we could not blame everything on a single virus. It seemed to me also that every living African, whether in good or ill health, is prey to many enemies of health that would interact one upon the other in many ways, within one human body. And thus I came to conclude that we have a desperate and pressing need to wage a war on all fronts to guarantee and realize the right of all our people to good health . . . One of the questions I have asked is: are safe sex, condoms, and antiretroviral drugs a sufficient response to the health catastrophe we face?'[5]

September 10, 2000: 'AIDS is a syndrome. It's a whole variety of diseases which affect a person because something negative has happened to the immune system. If the scientists come back and say this virus is part of the variety of things from which people acquire immune deficiency, I have no problem with that. But to say this is the sole cause, therefore the only response to it is antiretroviral drugs, I am saying we will never be able to solve the AIDS problem.'[6]

July 9, 2000: 'I believe that we should speak to one another honestly and frankly, with sufficient tolerance to respect everybody's point of view, with sufficient tolerance to allow all voices to be heard. Had we, as a people, turned our backs on these civilized precepts, we would never have achieved the much-acclaimed South African miracle of which all humanity is justly proud . . . [Yet] what I hear being said repeatedly, stridently, angrily, is – do not ask any questions!'[7]

What Mbeki is saying is really no different from what Dubos said 45 years ago or what Kunitz said 25 years later. All agree that there are etiologic agents – germs, for example – involved in causing disease, and that drugs are helpful in managing disease. Yet all affirm that this is not the whole story. Kunitz, the one MD of the group, a professor at an American medical school, even suggested that 'medical expertise may often be misapplied and even wrong in respect of the explanations it offers and treatments it recommends,' a suggestion comparable to what Mbeki had been saying. Kunitz's voice was not very loud in America but Mbeki's was very loud world-wide, and even louder because of the controversy. Yet instead of listening to Mbeki, the press mocked him. Instead of assuming he knew something about the public health of his own country, we lectured him from our own reductionist point of view. Instead of recognizing his contribution to enlarging *our* understanding of disease, we called him a quack.

When we don't listen to Mbeki, we – American medicine and the American people – are the losers. We have the money (for now) to pay for new diabetes drugs and new AIDS drugs, but focusing on drugs will not put a dent in either epidemic. We need to go back to Rene Dubos's classic work and to dig out Kunitz's obscure work. And then we need to listen humbly, with fresh ears, to the common sense coming from South Africa.

HEALING

CHAPTER NINE

Treatment

The healers are also confused, not about the aim of our work, but about the medicines we may use and about what may look like medicine but may end up being poison.

Ayi Kwei Armah, *The Healers*

In November 2000, the Nairobi *Sunday Nation* published an article on HIV/AIDS sympathetic to the views of South Africa's President Mbeki.[1] The article suggested that the main question facing all 'AIDS dissidents' such as Mbeki is 'Are we satisfied – or to what extent are we satisfied – with the answers which the scientific establishment has offered regarding HIV/AIDS medical theory and treatment?' Since I was the author of that article, I benefited from the feedback, including a long handwritten letter from a Nairobi AIDS dissident physician. He was not a traditional healer or 'witch doctor'; he was an African doctor trained in a Western-style medical school, and he knew Western medicine from the inside.

In his letter he made this general comment: 'In modern medicine we have developed some obsessions. Every disease **must** have a cause. It has to be a pathogen; if not, at least a gene! . . . The other obsession is, if found or imagined, a pathogen must be killed, at any cost . . .'[2] In accurately summarizing the foundations of modern scientific medicine, this doctor was able, with his outside–inside view, to see that our axioms can become obsessions. He knew that there is a lot more to disease than bugs and drugs. He also knew that antiretroviral chemotherapy for HIV/AIDS was not the definitive answer for AIDS, especially AIDS in Africa. He was able to see that there are larger questions than simply whether or not these expensive drugs reduce viral load.

SUFFERING AND HEALING IN AMERICA

Perhaps it is easier for people who have worked outside America to take a fresh look at American treatment options. The following vignettes all refer to drugs reviewed in 1998–99 issues of *The Medical Letter*, a biweekly medical publication that covers new drugs. The reviews commonly summarize the evidence for effectiveness of the new drug compared with the effectiveness of a placebo with no pharmacological properties. The patients are imaginary, but are very much like patients I have treated in America. I wrote the vignettes, however, while working in Africa.

Mary is a poor, overweight, middle-aged diabetic woman who has recently developed an ulcer on her leg. Regranex is a new topical drug, not yet on the drug list of her managed care plan. Almost half of the people who use it get complete healing; yet a quarter to a third of people with ulcers who use a placebo get complete healing. The drug costs $378 for the amount needed for healing. Should we call the managed care organization to plead for permission to use this drug?

Uncle Albert is 75 years old and has had painful knees from osteoarthritis for the past 10 years. A new drug, Hyaluronan, has resulted in decreased pain in half of the patients who had it injected in their knee. However, over a third had decreased pain with placebo saline injections, and nearly half felt similar relief with an oral non-steroidal anti-inflammatory drug, such as ibuprofen. The new drug costs $620, not covered by the insurance plan. Should I buy it for him?

A cousin in her late 30s has recently noticed increasing pain from her rheumatoid arthritis. Leflunomide, a new drug costing $1600 for six months' use, has resulted in 'some' (at least 20%) improvement at one year in almost half of the people who use it. However, a quarter to nearly a third of the people who use a placebo have the same subjective improvement. Disease progression by X-ray findings was at least four times more with a placebo than with the drug. Methotrexate, which she hasn't tried yet, also results in symptomatic improvement and slowed disease progression, though slightly less than the new drug; methotrexate costs about $300 for six months. Which drug should you advise her to use?

Ralph, an older brother in his mid 50s, has a desk job in an insurance company. He's had occasional chest pain for several years but just recently it became much more frequent, with minimal exertion, and his doctor diagnosed unstable angina. He has heard that at least 15% of people who are given heparin or a placebo will have a full myocardial infarction (heart attack) or die within 30 days. Two new drugs given immediately (Eptifibatide for $1625 or Tirofiban for $1260) can reduce his chance of heart attack or death by 1–3 percentage points. His insurance coverage is good. Should he use one of these drugs?

TREATMENT

A neighbor with long-standing diabetes has finally developed renal failure, and is being prepared for a kidney transplant. He has heard that with standard treatment to prevent rejection of the kidney graft, a third to a half of people will show symptoms of acute rejection by six months post-transplant. Graft survival at a year, though, is near 90%. One of two new expensive drugs (Daclizumab for $5855 or Basiliximab for $2448) can be added to the standard antirejection drugs, decreasing the acute rejection symptoms at six months to about one-fourth of people. Graft survival at a year is only a few percentage points higher. State funds do not cover these new drugs, and he is trying to raise money for them by a neighborhood campaign. Should you contribute?

George is dying from a very aggressive brain tumor (glioblastoma multiforme). He's just 48 and was operated on only last year, but the tumor has returned. The surgeon recommends that he re-operate and insert Gliadel wafers, which will slowly release the anticancer drug BCNU into the brain. In studies where a placebo was implanted, patients had a median survival of five months, and over half were dead at six months. With Gliadel treatment (which costs $12 480 for the drug alone), median survival was seven months, and over a third were dead at six months. George is rich, but miserable because he is unable to work and is in pain. Should he get the additional treatment?

Your sister has metastatic breast cancer. At 50 she found a breast mass, had surgery and chemotherapy, but two years later began having bone pain. Bone scans showed metastatic cancer. For the usual chemotherapy given at this stage of the disease, only a quarter of the patients respond; this response lasts almost half a year, and two-thirds are still alive a year after starting. There is a new drug, though, that can be added to the standard chemotherapy. Chemo plus Trastuzumab results in not quite half of the patients showing some response, which lasts three-fourths of a year. At the end of a year almost 80% are still alive, only 10% more than with standard chemotherapy, but all still have metastatic breast cancer. The new drug costs $13 575. Should she take it?

None of these stories mentions side effects, which every drug has. Only a few refer to standard, cheaper alternatives but in most situations they exist. In every case there is documented benefit from a placebo or from the original treatment that the new drug augments. In other words, there is evidence justifying the use of a placebo in every situation. There is also 'statistically significant' evidence that the new drug is better than a placebo in each case, though the difference in effect between baseline (no treatment) and placebo use is often greater than the difference between placebo and the new drug.

But since there is real, measurable benefit with all these drugs, is it ethical to consider the question of cost? In Africa, of course, it is unethical *not* to. But there is more than ethics involved. Does it make sense to use a marginally effective drug that will not really change the course of a disease? Are these drugs producing palliation or false hope? Does using them make sense in cultures where the concept of chronic disease has not yet been firmly established, as discussed in Chapter 7?

Since all of my patients are imaginary, I can influence what decisions they make. All of them found some additional information that pushed them to make some bold decisions. We have now really entered the world of fiction; I wish that these endings were as real as the situations.

Mary has been donating $10 of her welfare check monthly to a mission hospital. This amount pays for the whole drug treatment course of a child with meningitis. You mention to her that the new drug you're wondering about costs the same as treating 38 children with meningitis. She wants to know if there's any way you can get her drug, sell it, and use the money for the 38 children.

Uncle Albert has always felt a deep sense of justice in those arthritic bones. When you mention that the cost of the new injection would cover the surgeon's fee for three major cases in a rural African hospital, he asks for the saline injection.

Your cousin with rheumatoid arthritis is a complainer, but she is also grateful when she finds relief. You realize that the difference in cost between the new drug and methotrexate could pay two nurses' salaries for a year in the rural African hospital. You offer her the methotrexate.

In reading *National Geographic* magazine, Ralph finds out that very few people in rural Africa have his condition – that it's a disease of the developed world. He reads further and finds that very few people in rural Africa are covered by insurance, so that when they do get ill, they need to sell cows or land to cover their hospital bills. The price of one of the new drugs he was considering would buy two acres of agricultural land or cover a massive hospital bill. He uses the drug, but feels so guilty that he begins sending money to World Vision – after recovering from his coronary artery bypass graft surgery.

You discover that the amount your neighbor is trying to raise for minimal benefit in preventing graft rejection would cover the salary of a local doctor at a mission hospital for a year. You decide to decline contributing to his campaign.

George finds out that the cost of the drug his surgeon wants to implant in his brain would cover the entire hospital bills for over 30 very sick people at an African hospital, many of whom would be well on discharge. That same amount spent on him only delays the inevitable. He sees no reason to prolong his own suffering.

TREATMENT

Your sister is angry about her cancer – angry and depressed, because she loves life so much. Before marrying, she had worked briefly in Haiti and still remembers the laughter and joy she found there amid the squalor. She has discussed this with a woman she met during chemotherapy, also with metastatic breast cancer. They calculate that if the two of them decide to take the new drug, the amount of money they consume would run an entire mission hospital of 100 beds with a staff of 120 for a month. 'Though it seems crazy . . .' she tells you, she chooses the standard chemotherapy and saves every penny she can for a trip to that mission hospital before she dies.

CHAPTER TEN

Healing

Healing is work, not gambling. It is the work of inspiration, not manipulation. If we the healers are to do the work of helping to bring our people together again, we need to know such work is the work of a community. It cannot be done by any individual. It should not depend on any single person however heroic he may be. And it can't be done by people who don't understand the healing vocation – no matter how good such people may be as individuals.

Ayi Kwei Armah, *The Healers*

In this chapter I want to talk about healing and how it differs from treating. **Healing** means being made whole; 'wholeness' and 'health' share the same Greek root word. **Treating** is doing something to arrest a disease. Healing has a broad focus and looks for a certain result: 'wholeness.' Treating has a narrower focus – a particular disease – and looks for a narrower result – getting rid of the disease. I will use my experience as a framework for this chapter, especially in light of my own recent retreat from the activities of healing to those of treating.

One of the reasons I chose to study family medicine was because I wanted to learn about healing. Family medicine, as I understood it, was a way to coordinate the advances of American medicine after World War II. But even more, it was a response to, and a reaction against, the depersonalizing and compartmentalizing effects of those advances. By the end of the 1960s technology and specialized medicine had increased so much that not only was primary care at risk, healing itself was as well. Family medicine was more than just a way to upgrade the old GPs and give them respectability in an environment where board examinations were more and more important. It was a return to seeing a patient not just as a bag of organs but as a 'whole person' living in a family which could contribute to a disease and also influence its outcome. I felt family medicine would give me the opportunity to study, in Paul Tournier's phrase, 'the healing of persons.'[1]

Implicit in my thinking was this: specialized technical medicine was becoming very good at fine-tuning the diagnosis of disease, as well as treating those micro diagnoses. I had respect for those treatments, but sensed that treatment was not always accompanied by healing.[2] I knew people could be 'cured' yet not 'made whole.' I even knew people who were 'whole' – i.e. content, well integrated, and healthy – even though they had a condition or disease that hadn't been cured. In other words, I knew that though there was an important overlap between treatment and healing, they weren't the same thing. My hope was that family medicine training could give me an overview of treatment skills, while at the same time showing me how to use them for healing.

At least now, looking back, that's what I would want from a family medicine program. At the time, I think I assumed that simply by mastering the primary treatment skills of all the specialties, including psychiatry, and by offering them to everyone in the family, I'd have a better shot at healing. I think 30 years ago my program assumed the same thing, and they gave me that overview.

We did not talk much about 'healing,' though. Family medicine was only seven years old then and it was important in that first generation to define the curriculum and gain academic credibility, all in terms that the medical establishment understood. But we weren't outsiders trying to get in, we were the medical establishment. So naturally, we built family medicine in terms we understood: technical diagnosis and treatment terms, not 'healing' terms. To us, then, adequate diagnosis and treatment *were* healing.

Let me add here, parenthetically, that medicine does not have, nor should it have, a monopoly on healing. There are many 'healing arts,' many professionals involved with helping people become whole. We in family medicine understand especially the approach of other scientists, i.e. social scientists such as psychologists and social workers. But we dare not delegate to them the entire task of making people whole. Their sphere of influence is almost as narrow as ours. Pastors and spiritual directors can have a very deep influence in helping some people become whole – but only some people. Wise friends and relatives can be remarkable healers – but only some friends and relatives. Actors, singers, and writers can profoundly affect a journey toward wholeness – sometimes. Even an entire culture can be one that encourages either health and wholeness or disease and fragmentation.

But if medicine is one of the healing arts, how intentional are we in helping our patients become whole? Are we satisfied with diagnosing and treating the biomedical parts of their disease and letting counselors and pastors help them live with, or fight off, the disease? And do all of our treatments aid in healing or could some of them actually be counterproductive in bringing wholeness? I shall return to this shortly.

When I completed my family medicine training I began practicing in Maynardville, the county seat of Union County, Tennessee. There my wife (also a doctor) and I worked in what might be called an ideal place for family medicine. We saw entire families and provided them with the whole range of outpatient services, admitting them to St Mary's Hospital in Knoxville for inpatient care. We lived in the community and occasionally made home visits, so we saw our patients' disease in its context. As medical examiner and jail doctor, I even had an inside look at the seamier side of life in Union County. We worked closely with the Cherokee mental health system, and so had immediate access to professional counselors. Our first employer was the Public Health Department, giving us an official link there. We were not just 'organ doctors' or 'body doctors'; we weren't even restricted to being 'family doctors.' We were, in some senses, 'community doctors.'

In all of this activity, were we involved in healing? It's not a question I asked at the time. Mostly we treated our patients and were happy when they 'got better.' I was taken then by the ideas of 'community health' more than 'the healing of persons' but I think we did do more than just treat; I think we did try to heal. Beyond the three-ring circus of services we provided or arranged for, we entered some people's lives. We struggled with them as they tried to get rid of an affliction or, more often, to live sanely with it. Here and there and now and then, sometimes because of all the 'ancillary' services and sometimes relying on techniques we'd been taught, but often using only the personality and common sense God gave us, we worked to help people become whole.

Then after seven years, we left to work in Africa. There were many reasons, most unrelated to our work as healers because 'the healing of persons' was not in the center of what we did. But our leaving did give us a chance to take a fresh look at family medicine, and indirectly at healing.

Family medicine intended to provide cradle to grave, minor to serious, medical and surgical healthcare for everyone in the family – or at least to 'orchestrate' that care. The idea was that such a broad view would reduce fragmentation of services by having them better coordinated, with a single manager or 'tour guide' through these services. Underneath, I think, was the hope that this single manager would be in a better position to help the patient heal.[3]

However, our experience was different. Instead of 'coordinating' care, we found ourselves squeezed between the minor and serious. The increasing standard of care required that, for most of our hospitalized patients, we consult specialists and they tended to take control of the patient care. We didn't orchestrate, we listened. And with the other 'end' of care, the common minor conditions, we found that nurse practitioners and physician's assistants did an excellent job in caring for these patients. Sometimes they did even better than we did because, frankly, we eventually found some of that work boring. We were still the tour guides through our circus of caring services, but healing and wholeness became more elusive.

I mentioned above that I was 'taken' by the ideas of community health, suggesting that I was in a 'phase' that I would eventually 'get over.' That doesn't quite get it. It's true that my first job in Africa was mostly in community health, and that I do not have the same involvement in community health as I used to. But the healing of communities is not a phase; I think it is an integral part in the healing of persons.

What I found difficult was to do both at the same time and so for a while I did only community health. My experience was like that of a nephrologist being asked to care for someone with renal failure who also had heart disease and significant emotional and family problems resulting from the diseases. To accurately diagnose and prescribe for the kidney disease requires one set of skills; to care for the patient's emotional and social problems requires a different attitude and different set of skills. Likewise, the healing of persons requires a different attitude and set of skills from the healing of communities.

I see that now. But first in Union County and then in Africa, my question was less 'which set of skills do I have?' than 'which task is more important?' or rather 'which task is more important to me now?' I knew that prevention, or maintaining health, was preferable to trying to repair it once it had been disturbed. I felt too that the restoring of health had a better chance of being effective when people in the community were involved in the process. Any healing, I thought, should be the offering of a remedy and the active reception of that remedy. Passive recipients, whether individuals or communities, may be cured but only active recipients could be healed. That belief led me not just to the discipline of public health but to the approach called community health.

Community health, however, proved far more difficult than I first envisioned. Perhaps that is only a reflection of the difficulty of any healing. There are plenty of public health remedies – vaccinations, public pipes or private latrines, homemade rehydration solutions for diarrhea, mosquito nets, and so on – but more often than not, we impose these remedies on communities. More often than not, people are passive rather than active recipients. More often than not, communities are 'cured' of their health hazards without being made whole.

Gradually we let go of community health; more and more in Africa we were asked to practice 'individual' medicine. And as we did, we discovered that two things were happening to us: we were getting better at the craft of medicine, and we were no longer attempting to heal. Each requires some explanation.

Western scientific medicine in Africa is, in some ways, the medicine of Osler: the careful use of history and physical examination to diagnose illness. It is in other ways the medicine of the American 1950s and 1960s: basic X-ray and laboratory to aid diagnosis, and basic medicine and surgery to treat most conditions. It is, of course, also the medicine of the 1990s: there are CT scanners and fiber-optic scopes and subspecialty surgery available in big cities, and even small rural mission hospitals have ultrasound machines and, sometimes, the newer drugs.

But in much of the Third World there are no automated blood chemistry machines, no ventilators, no renal dialysis, no intensive care units, no medical or surgical subspecialists. Family doctors and general surgeons – but often just 'GPs' – are the end of the line and mostly see only referrals from physician assistant- or nurse-level primary providers. Far from being 'squeezed' for work by boredom on the one side and specialists on the other, family doctors *are* the specialists but without the technology of American specialists. And without the expectations America lays on them.

The result is that we must rely more on our hands and ears and eyes for diagnosis, and that we must treat with ingenuity. Cost-consciousness is not a style of practice that can be rewarded by an HMO; it is the only way to practice. African medicine and surgery rely far less on technology simply because it's not there. Yet the amazing thing is how often we can diagnose accurately and treat adequately without high technology. We become better clinicians, even by Western standards, precisely because we lack the technology characteristic of Western medicine.

After some time of practicing this medicine in both Tanzania and Kenya, I began to think about what had been obvious all along: that I was not building long-term relationships with my patients. I was like an American surgeon or ICU nurse: I got to know the sickest patients very well while they were ill but then they would either die or go home, and often I would not see them again. Most of the poor health in Africa is from acute infections or trauma; little is chronic and degenerative, as in America. I was not building long-term relationships with people because of the nature of their disease and my role as the one being referred to. I was doing more extensive diagnosis and treatment than in America but was no longer thinking about long-term therapy and change . . . or healing.

And, in a way, I didn't have to. I may have been the 'end of the line' for Western medicine but no one saw Western medicine as the end of the line. People came to our hospitals for 'treatment' without, I think, ever expecting 'healing.' Healing was still a matter for traditional healers and culture and family. Even the bulk of Africans who had joined a religion from 'outside' – Islam or Christianity – saw in that religion the ultimate provider of healing. Doctors are viewed as craftsmen, not artists; as technicians, not healers.

To say it another way: more is expected of each doctor because there are fewer doctors, but less is expected from the profession as a whole. We are expected to be good technicians, as in America, but we are not expected to be able to prevent every death. A bad outcome in America means a lawsuit because there is nothing beyond medicine when medicine fails. A bad outcome in Africa is a tragedy with spiritual, not legal, implications. There is always something beyond medicine and for that reason, we are not expected to heal, but only to treat.

Now we must return to American family medicine and ask whether or not my original expectation – to learn about healing in a family medicine training program – was reasonable.

To summarize the problem: American subspecialty technological medicine is very good at diagnosing and treating, but has been accused of neglecting the 'whole person.' More than this: the more a healthcare system uses technology, the less it depends on human or 'natural' resources for healing. It can even suppress 'natural' healing in the same way that continued high doses of corticosteroids can suppress the 'natural' production of endogenous corticosteroids.[4] But the biggest effect of high-technology medicine is that by focusing on biomedical treatment, it ignores the question of healing altogether.

Scientific medicine in Africa, on the other hand, employs less powerful technology and has not yet eliminated the healing forces of the culture. Therefore, when scientific medicine in Africa ignores the question of healing, as does its American counterpart, the consequences are very different. The treatment paradigm is the same, but it is at work in an entirely different culture.

American family medicine intended to address the problem of fragmentation by asking one cadre of doctors to oversee healthcare for the entire family: to recommend preventive activities, diagnose and treat the majority of their illnesses, and efficiently connect them with the correct technology and specialists for more complicated disease. The assumption was that proper training in common illnesses, together with a broad understanding of what 'high-tech' medicine can offer, would provide a doctor with the tools necessary for complete treatment, which was assumed to be the same as healing.

But the third decade of family medicine took a twist that we didn't expect, though perhaps we should have. The 'high-tech' medicine that we coordinate is very expensive and we long ago chose to not let that be a factor in deciding whether and when to use that technology. It was a matter of ethics: life and health were at stake and we could not endorse a lesser level of health, or at least treatment, based merely on money. We would offer – or 'prescribe' – the best to everyone and it was up to the patient, or the insurance company or the government, to find the money to pay for it.

They did – for a while. And in the process, 'they' gained control of our medical system. Now they have told us there is simply not enough money to pay for all the latest technology for everyone, so they – the ones who pay – have changed the way we practice. And since their concern is economic, their changes are based on economics. The healing versus treating debate disappears from the agenda.

For family medicine, the change is this: we first became a specialty, in part, to reduce fragmentation and treat the whole person. Now we are being told that we are 'gate-keepers,' suggesting that real treatment occurs only inside the gate. We originally were given extra training so that we could do more than 'general practitioners' and treat patients without referring them. Now we are given extra training in diagnostic procedures so we can treat patients *by* referring them. The focus is shifting from treating the whole patient to navigating that patient through the whole medical system.

This does not mean that we no longer treat patients. But it does mean that our center of gravity is changing, and what is distinctive about us as a specialty is different from what it used to be. Thirty years ago, we were developing the expertise to manage clinical problems in the huge 'overlap' area of body, mind, and family. Now we are more able to select out those few patients in this overlap needing 'definitive' organic treatment but less able, it seems, to manage the whole problem. The fallout for healing is obvious.

But then again, is it fair to ask family medicine to attempt what neither African nor American scientific medicine does? Can any scientific curative system be expected to help make people whole, especially when the culture they come from is fractured? Is healthcare really the sphere for healing?

It's a difficult question. If healing is the business of family medicine, we need to make major changes in our curriculum, recruit a different kind of new doctor, and try to reclaim what Western medicine lost centuries ago. On the other hand, if healing is beyond the scope of family medicine, then family medicine is off the hook – and all of American medicine is on the rack, tortured by a people in need of healing and seeking it from a system set up only to cure.

I read the last half of this chapter to my wife, who squirmed until I came to the last few paragraphs. I had been asking the wrong question all along, she said, hoping for family medicine to teach me how to heal. Of course medicine can't heal, she said. She, a board-certified pediatrician who also passed the boards for family medicine, a 'generalist' who can untwist a compound volvulus, do a bowel resection and primary anastomosis and have the patient well and home in less than 10 days – she said without hesitation, 'Only God can heal.'

Now, how can we convince the American public?

CHAPTER ELEVEN

Family medicine

You are slowly dying under the weight of evidence . . . Evidence is a quality of the surface. Your science is a triumph of evidence, a proliferation of the surface. It makes you masters of the external, but at the same time it exiles you there, more and more.

Cheikh Hamidou Kane, *Ambiguous Adventure*

I wrote these reflections in Africa nearly 10 years ago, after spending a year in America when managed care was the new demonic savior. Recently, I spent three more years practicing family medicine in a place where managed care did not bother me, Indian Health Service. Unfortunately, I found little difference in the crises enumerated below, except a more open admission that we need to re-evaluate ourselves and consider the future of family medicine. But nothing fundamentally has changed. Today I would add that we are also in a prevention crisis, the subject of the next chapter.

American family medicine – this same family medicine that I studied hoping to learn about healing – is in a crisis. The odd thing is that we don't seem to know it. Managed care has come and we still practice medicine. Costs are spiraling but we still practice medicine. The business of 'alternative' healing is booming and we still practice medicine. Technology performs wizardry but we still practice medicine. Medical ethics committees intrude in our practice but we still practice medicine. We prefer to view all these changes around us as challenges, or some even as allies, that don't affect the essence of who we are. We are willing to evolve, and that is what we hope is the result of these changes. It just does not seem that we are tottering on any knife-edge or are faced with any single critical decision.

We *are* on a knife-edge and we are faced with some critical decisions. It is even possible that family medicine may be unrecognizable in another generation, at least to those who envisioned the modern specialty of family medicine built on the foundation of the old general practice. Now change is not necessarily bad, if the new family medicine is what we have chosen it to be. And that is exactly the point: there are several choices confronting us and that is why we are in a crisis. Knowing that we are in a crisis is the first step to surviving it.

But we are not in *just one* crisis. There are several forces outside ourselves that are squeezing us and these forces have precipitated at least five crises for family medicine, each with specific questions and each with consequences of not facing the questions. We are in an identity crisis (who are we?), a vision crisis (what do we do?), a financial crisis (how do we do it?), a methodological crisis (how do we know what to do?), and an ethical crisis (how do we decide what to do?). And although these crises may overlap, we don't often think of them together, which is one of the reasons why it is difficult to realize that we are in crisis. We may view each alone as only a challenge, because each alone will not destroy us. Together they might.

Identity crisis

When I was a family medicine resident in the mid-1970s, the metaphor that we were offered for ourselves was that of orchestra director. We were not expected to play all the instruments but we needed to know the score and to coordinate the players. The presence of so much technology and so many specialists in medicine meant that 'whole person' medicine was at risk of vanishing and we wanted to rescue it.

It was a good metaphor because it was a good idea. The problem is that the metaphor didn't work in practice. The other players weren't asking for a director. Instead of coordinating care, family medicine found itself in competition with other 'primary care' specialties. That was because the metaphor had changed. We were no longer seen as directors of an orchestra but, as noted in the previous chapter, keepers of a gate.

It was we in family medicine who created the orchestra director metaphor. But it is the insurance companies and managed care plans who have pushed the gate-keeper metaphor. They understandably want to control what they pay *inside* the gate, and so looked for providers who could treat some conditions less expensively *outside* and limit who gets inside. While the role is a reasonable one, the shift in metaphor is troubling. It suggests that real medical care is specialist care ('inside') and it reduces the possibility that family medicine could have any humanizing influence on that care.

But more importantly, we have accepted the new metaphor. We are surrounded by plenty of specialists who are happy to provide care 'inside' and the managed care plans make it more financially attractive for us to stay 'outside.'

We like being gate-keepers; many of us don't even admit our own patients to the hospital any more.

Have we adequately examined this new metaphor? We carry with us beliefs in 'comprehensiveness' and 'continuity': can we maintain these beliefs as gate-keepers? Are we ready to let go of the influence that we thought we could have on specialty-dominated technological medicine? And even more to the point, can we survive as gate-keepers? If we can treat the minor conditions less expensively than specialists, while selectively ushering the sickest people through the gate, can't nurse practitioners and physician's assistants do this even more cheaply?

We at the end of this first generation of family medicine are having an identity crisis. That is a normal part of growing up. We are under no obligation to follow all the dreams of our leaders in the 1960s and 1970s. However, as we change, it is important that we have reasons for what we are becoming, that we are in control of the metaphors that we are following. It is important that we know we are having an identity crisis, so we can choose what we will become.

Vision crisis

Similar to the identity crisis of who we *are*, we are in a vision crisis of what we see our goals to be, of what we *do*. As with the identity crisis, our vision crisis has developed slowly and is best seen by comparing ourselves with family medicine of 30 years ago.

During my family medicine training, faculty were beginning to talk about the 'bio-psychosocial model' of healthcare. We were beginning to feel that we had a unique approach to people's disease that included far more than laboratory tests, medications, and procedures. We were committed to mastering the basics of this standard medical care, but also of filling in the gaps that specialist technological medicine left. We were determined not to be just half-baked internists and pediatricians but, by our approach, to be a new kind of specialist.

The condition that epitomized this new approach was the various 'somat-ization syndromes' – psychosomatic conditions that cause troubling physical symptoms with no organic basis that we could find. For most medical and psychiatric conditions, there was some specialist we could refer to if we were unable to diagnose or treat adequately. But we were the end of the line for somatization syndromes. Our patients saw no need to go to psychiatrists because they felt their problem was in their body. Yet medical specialists could only order more complicated investigations which 'ruled out' organic disease but did nothing to treat the condition. We began to learn techniques to manage these conditions, never expecting to 'cure' them but hopefully, as with any chronic, incurable condition, to provide some relief.

It's not that we wanted to be specialists for only one disease, though psychosomatic conditions are extremely common and need someone's expertise. Somatization simply illustrates how we were trying to approach all disease in a different, more 'wholistic' way. We may not have been the end of the line for diabetes care but we were willing to be the place where the buck stopped, the end of the line, for the *person* who had diabetes.

We still, in family medicine, would like to be our patient's main advocate in the medical system. But we seem to have lost something – something, perhaps, we never really had. Our teachers in family medicine must sometimes be specialists and we cannot help but absorb their 'biomedical' approach. The best of us learn to integrate the 'bio' part from specialists with the 'psychosocial' part we learn elsewhere. But too often these parts remain unconnected and too often, our necessary contact with the rest of the medical community reinforces only our biomedical part.

The fallout for family medicine is this: we are learning more and more procedures (especially diagnostic procedures, enabling us to be better gate-keepers) but we are beginning to forget how to heal. We have been so influenced by the specialists who taught us the procedures that we have begun to equate curing with healing. In trying to apprehend all that technology offers to cure, we have fewer opportunities to help our patients bear under their affliction, to help them suffer.

What is our vision? Is our goal to help people heal? Is our goal to provide first-contact primary care and identify the people who need specialist care? Or is our goal to survive as one of the primary care specialties by offering the services that managed care wants us to offer – and will pay us well for? We may likely affirm all these goals and therein lies the crisis, for each goal will lead in a different direction. We should recognize this as a crisis and confront the questions that the crisis raises.

Financial crisis

The next crisis, that of spiraling healthcare costs, is one we in family medicine share with all of medicine. However, we 'own' this crisis even less than those above, because we have been personally squeezed very little by it. True, insurance plans may limit what drugs we can prescribe for their patients or erect barriers to how we plan to work up their patients. But we see these as irritations, not critiques of the way we practice medicine. Our salaries have not fallen in family medicine; we are not personally having a financial crisis.

Healthcare is. The US spends 14% of its gross national product on healthcare; many European countries with similar or better health statistics spend just over half that. Our insurance carriers, including the government, are saying that 14% is too much. So far the result has been more restrictions and more paperwork but we have not challenged our 'standard,' and therefore *amount*, of care.

Can our economy afford to continue spending disproportionately on one sector, especially without corresponding results? Isn't it possible that if we don't change how we practice, we will one day be confronted with radical rationing by those who pay? That rationing may take the form of limiting who gets healthcare but it could also take the form of limiting who gets paid. Then the financial crisis could be ours personally. Isn't it better to confront it now?

There are many reasons why America spends so much on medical care; I'd like to consider just one. If our identity, who we are, has been challenged by managed care and what we do has been influenced by specialists, then how we do it (and how much we spend) is determined by technology. We follow the current technology-based 'standard of care' because we feel we must – but often also because we believe in it.

Consider this: one day, when I was working in Sudan, I began to feel weak and sore in my joints. Later that day, when I went outside to the latrine, I noticed my urine was golden orange in color. I went inside and went to bed to begin my recovery from hepatitis. Shortly thereafter, I became visibly jaundiced and felt like there was a brick under my right rib cage. I was unable to work for a couple of weeks and a month later had still not regained all my strength. I had no laboratory tests performed on myself and took no medications. I recovered fully and when I returned to the US, a cousin who worked for a laboratory company offered to do blood work, which confirmed hepatitis A.

I had a major illness which cost me several weeks off work but I purchased nothing from the healthcare system. It's not that I don't believe in technology. I have benefited from appropriate technology for several other illnesses in Africa: a slit lamp and antiviral drugs for corneal ulcers; a urinalysis and Cipro for pyelonephritis; insecticide-treated bed nets, blood smears, and antimalarials for prevention and treatment of malaria. I recovered fully from all these conditions and the cost for my diagnosis and treatment was far less than it would have been in America.

Medical care in the US does not need to be as expensive as it is. Bed and board in our hospital in Kenya is $7.00 a day. We use quality generic medications. A man hospitalized with bacterial pneumonia will probably be charged under $100 and will recover as well as if he received treatment in the US. A woman with a C-section will likely have a bill of under $500 and most of the time, the outcome will be what she could expect in America. Of course, we cannot offer MRI scans and cardiac surgery but the patient with pneumonia or placenta previa doesn't mind.

Our entire 'standard' has gotten so high that we apply it everywhere, even where we know a 'lower' – and cheaper – standard would be equally effective. In fact, an equally effective standard would not be lower at all. As family physicians, we have worked hard to be competent in the diagnostic and therapeutic technology available for primary care. We should be working equally hard to know when it is not necessary, and when it can actually inhibit healing. Newer, more 'accurate' tests are not always necessary; neither are newer, more powerful drugs. Yet both are undoubtedly more expensive.

The financial crisis in medicine is presenting us with some choices. There are clearly risks in not facing these choices. It rings hollow to say that technology is beyond our control, that we are bound by this expensive standard of care. Technology is in *our* control: *we* order the tests and treatments. And by so doing, *we* set the standard of care. How we determine that standard brings us to the next crisis.

Methodology crisis

We have looked at who we are, what we do, and how we do it. Now we should look at how we know what to do, what methods we use to choose which diagnostics and therapeutics are really effective and integral to our standard of care. The critical issue here is evidence-based medicine.

In one sense this is not a crisis at all. Just as, 30 years ago, the bio-psychosocial model was the new kid on the block, now evidence-based medicine is. And as the bio-psychosocial model was in some ways not at all new but made explicit what many healers had known by intuition, so evidence-based medicine articulates what we thought we were doing all along: basing our decisions on scientific evidence. The surprise is in how much of our medicine is not evidence based – and that's where the crisis comes from.

We do much of what we do because it 'makes sense': we order tests to rule in or out what might be there; we order treatments that seem to counter the pathology that we find. But how many of these diagnostics and therapeutics have been proven in controlled studies to do what we hope they are doing? How many screening tests pick up early treatable forms of disease as dependably as Pap smears? What is the ultimate outcome of fetal monitoring? How many antihypertensive drugs have been proven to decrease mortality? What evidence is there that a CT scan is useful in the work-up of a headache? Is there any proof that routine pre-operative care for elective surgery should always include a chest X-ray, EKG, CBC, blood chemistries, and urinalysis?

Evidence-based medicine could do wonders to rein in technology, to make our standard of care truly science based, and to reduce the cost of healthcare. The crisis occurs in family medicine when we choose not to look at the evidence and not to listen to it. If our medicine is not evidence based, what is it based on?

There is, however, another side to this story. Mature evidence-based advocates are the first to admit that lack of 'conclusive' evidence for a procedure or drug does not automatically invalidate its use. Studies have not been done to test everything that we do. Patients have disease and they ask us for relief. Our treatments may not reduce mortality (the ultimate 'evidence') and they may not always work but if the patients are relieved, were we wrong to prescribe in good faith what had not been 'proven'?

Medicine is still an art as well as a science, and family medicine above all must know this, for we never deal just with organs that we palpate and biopsy but people to whom we relate. Family medicine must keep one foot in science and the other in art. Our methodology must maintain its links with science and 'evidence' but we should never forget our common sense and our obligation to be *with* our patients, especially when we have no evidence. The crisis in family medicine is not evidence-based medicine; the crisis is when we forget that we must have reasons for what we do. Or, worse still, when we choose only evidence or only intuition.

Ethical crisis

When family medicine was born, we did not have a lot of confusion about medical ethics; we were not in a crisis. As described in Chapter 5, most family physicians made decisions based on what they thought was best for the patient. We used our own values and our intuition to make thorny decisions. But as technology increased and as patients became better informed, we found that intuition was not enough. Medical ethics grew as a discipline and made clear that the values and intuition of the doctor were an inadequate basis for decision making in a pluralist society. Patient autonomy, they said, should be the foundation. There were no universal answers to the increasingly difficult questions. Each of us is a free, responsible individual who should be intimately involved with decisions about his or her healthcare.

We agree; we'll respect autonomy. But when we do, we precipitate for ourselves the ethical crisis, because technological medicine does not easily adapt itself to consumer autonomy. Modern medicine is complicated, with some areas incomprehensible even to other doctors. Making intelligent choices, or even asking intelligent questions, can require a great deal of basic knowledge. Beyond this, patients confronted with choices are often frightened, anxious or angry because of their illness; they may not be in a frame of mind to reflect on options. They may not even at that point want the autonomy that society insists they have. Physicians are then caught between 'respecting' autonomy and leaving the patient alone, or being directive and risking paternalism. It is not just a question of bedside manner, it is an illustration of an ethical crisis.

We cannot deny that autonomy is pivotal in our culture and needs to be recognized in healthcare. But we also must remember that physicians have often helped patients not because they honored their autonomy but because they cared for them and had compassion on them. We cannot ignore patient autonomy but we must remember that it is a two-edged sword. Autonomy can lead to independence or isolation and responsibility can be a privilege or a burden, especially to people who are confronting a major illness.

The ethical crisis brings us back to the core of who we are as family physicians. If our bottom line is to enter into relationships with our patients that result in their being healed, we need to take their autonomy seriously. But we also need to trust our common sense, to recognize that autonomy itself can be a cause of anomie and malaise, that the very philosophical foundation of our culture can be the cause of much of our disease. We cannot ignore the autonomy of our patients but we dare not worship it. We can no longer assume that our own values are universal but we dare not ignore the compassion those values produce in us. We are indeed on a knife edge.

Family medicine is in crisis. Crisis originally meant the decisive moment or turning point in the course of a disease, when it becomes clear whether the patient will recover or die. Family medicine will not likely die but it will also not likely return to being what the leaders of the 1960s and 1970s envisioned it to be. The crises suggested here present us with several issues that we need to grapple with. Our only problem will be ignoring them.

PREVENTION

CHAPTER TWELVE

Prevention – 1

In the water the gazer saw a world in which some, a large number, had a prevalent disease. The disease was an urge to fragment everything. And the disease gave infinite satisfaction to the diseased, because it gave them control.

Ayi Kwei Armah, *The Healers*

Near the beginning of this study (Chapter 4), we looked at several characters from Greek mythology who still represent for us facets of modern Western healthcare. There were Aesculapius, representing healing by medicine, and Prometheus, representing technology. We also met Chiron, the centaur who might represent the humility that could be an antidote to our hubris. Now we must consider Hygeia.

Hygeia was the guardian of health. Such an important role would be thought to generate a lot of stories but classical Greek mythology says little about Hygeia. Even her origin is obscure. Some accounts say she was a daughter of Aesculapius; others suggest that she was 'a concept rather than a historical person remembered from the myths of their past'; 'an emanation, a personification of Athena, the goddess of reason.'[1] We can understand why some questioned her descent from Aesculapius; we can connect better with her sisters Panakeia (panacea), or 'cure-all,' and Iaso, the goddess of recovery, the Healer.

Today, we still have trouble placing or even defining 'health' in our panoply of medical care. We too think maintaining health has something to do with reason or common sense but common sense is not a medical discipline. We'd prefer our guardian of health to stay in the Aesculapian family, so our Hygeia is called 'prevention,' which today is most definitely a sister of Panakeia and Iaso. And she is becoming more and more like them.

We certainly take prevention seriously. It is part of most physicians' work today, more than it has ever been. There are more and more vaccines. We learn how to put tubes in increasing numbers of orifices to look for early treatable forms of disease. We use more and more medicines to treat pre-symptomatic forms of disease. And we increasingly must play our role in health education: the dispensing of good advice that, if our well patients would only follow it, would keep them from being sick patients.

We can, in other words, try to prevent a disease before it occurs (primary prevention), catch it at an early treatable stage (secondary prevention) or even treat the full-blown disease well to reduce morbidity and mortality (tertiary prevention). Where should the emphasis of our healthcare system be? Where should doctors focus their attention?

The obvious answer is that all three approaches are needed. The practical answer for primary care doctors is that secondary prevention – screening and treating pre-symptomatic disease – is the most appropriate role, or at least the role that merges most naturally into the doctor–patient relationship. Unfortunately, for many Western physicians, all prevention has come to be equated with this *secondary* prevention, even though screening and treating pre-symptomatic disease is only a small part of all of prevention. This reductionism precipitates several ethical questions, illustrated by the following story.

J and S are in their late 40s and have an eight-year-old daughter, K. They live in surburban Ohio. In the last several years, S has had routine mammography several times, leading to three breast biopsies. All were negative. J donates blood and was told that on routine screening, his blood tested positive for one of the HIV viruses – type 3. A further test was indeterminate. J and S have had no exposure to AIDS. S's blood was tested and a year later she had received only the bill, but no result. A few years ago K had an eye problem. Her parents took her to a specialist who examined her, did a blood test, and said that she would one day develop rheumatoid arthritis. They see the specialist with K several times a year and K still has no signs of systemic disease. Her eye is doing well.

J and S are responsible people, wanting to protect their health. They have obeyed the recommendations of our healthcare system, carried out by doctors trying to provide them with the current standard of care. But they still don't know if one of S's biopsies will eventually be positive or what J's 'indeterminate' blood test means or whether K will ever get ill and, if so, what that will involve. Even though all three are 'healthy' – they have no symptoms, no 'chief complaints' – yet all three are 'patients,' unsure that they have good health, unwillingly hooked in to our medical system.

No one in this story acted out of excess fear; no one acted unethically. However, the story of J, S and K raises several questions about 'preventive medicine,'[2] similar to the questions we raised about chronic disease treatment at the end of Chapter 7.

Are those who participate in screening aware of the 'positive predictive value' of the screening tests used – that is, the likelihood that a positive test really means the person tested has the disease? With most tests, there is not a complete correlation between a positive test and having the disease. The test may be positive even though the patient doesn't have the disease (a 'false positive') and this happens more often when many people are screened in a population in which the incidence of that disease is low. The nature of screening is that people with negative tests are usually reassured but told to return at a future date for a repeat test. People with positive tests are 'followed up' with further tests, which sometimes contradict the first test. The physician may be reassured by the second negative test but the patient is often left wondering why that first test was positive.

Have we confronted the emotional impact of that false-positive test? Unless a condition can be labeled with a 'diagnosis,' we don't consider it as a 'disease'; we view reactive stress only as part of the 'real' condition we're treating. Since reacting with stress to a false-positive test is not a 'real' disease, we don't know what to do with it other than 'reassure' once a second more accurate test is negative. Yet *we* caused the stress and reassurance this time does not assure that the *next* screening test will be negative. One effect of widespread screening is increased stress and apprehension in the entire population.

When we prescribe 'preventive medicines,' are we aware of the 'number needed to treat' (NNT) in order to help one person? Historically in scientific medicine, we would like our intervention to be successful most of the time – or at least half the time (NNT = 2). With preventive drugs today, however, we accept much less effective medicines (NNT = 30 or 50 or even 100). For example, in treating otherwise healthy people with high cholesterol, 'the trial of pravastatin for primary prevention by WOSCOP (the West of Scotland Coronary Prevention Study) would indicate that of 10 000 patients treated with a statin for five years, 9755 would receive no benefit.'[3] Yet Western medicine now says this is not only acceptable but is the standard of care. We can of course celebrate the better health of the 245 but have we been honest about the cost? Beyond the monetary cost of treating over 9000 people for the benefit of just over 200, there are the side effects of the drugs and the transformation of 9000 healthy people into patients dependent on the medical system.

Is probability an appropriate science for individual patients? We base decisions about screening (and much else in medicine, from treatment of hyperlipidemia to chemotherapy for cancer) on probability. When the unit of study is a whole community, this makes sense and of course, individual people are members of whole communities. But as physicians, we are faced with individuals. The use of a certain screening test (or treatment modality) may have been shown in large studies to cause a few percent improvement in people's health – statistically significant, of course. But does our individual patient *want* to undergo this test or treatment, knowing that the chance of personal benefit is really quite small?

How much of our passion for screening and treating risk factors is rooted in modern medicine's desire to control? We control the conditions surrounding birth (to make it 'safe'), control the course of an illness, control the moment of death – and now with screening, are we trying to control the future? In screening asymptomatic people, and especially in treating asymptomatic 'conditions' (hypercholesterolemia, hypertension, menopause, decreasing bone density, abnormal pap smears, etc.), we have helped to prevent advanced forms of disease – the same as we have made childbirth safer with hospital births and kept people alive longer with intensive care for terminal conditions. These accomplishments give us the illusion of control, reinforced by each 'success.' However, things still can go awry at a hospital birth, the person with the terminal condition eventually dies, and some people who screened negative for a disease still develop it. We all *know* that we don't have ultimate control over life and death but we still would like to have it. Have we, and our patients, begun to think that screening is actually a way to know and control our futures?

Some of these questions arise because we have chosen to keep Hygeia in the family of Aesculapius. She has learned pharmacology from her sister Panakeia, the drug goddess, and in doing so has begun to lose the reason that linked her with Athena. This does not mean, however, that we are rejecting primary prevention and its reasonableness. On the contrary, we medical people are trying to offer what we can to *help*. And what we are offering is that all people, both sick and well, become permanent patients, dependent on us and our medical system to know whether or not they are healthy, and dependent on us to stay that way.

'It is not the healthy who need the doctor, but the sick.' All three synoptic Gospels carry these words of Jesus. In His day, this was obvious. He was using an observation no one would debate to make a spiritual point, that He had come not for the virtuous but for sinners. Today His observation of the medical system is no longer obvious. Is it no longer true?

CHAPTER THIRTEEN

Prevention – 2

> The public entrusts [medicine-men] with the duty of removing what may harm the community.
>
> John S Mbiti, *African Religions and Philosophy*

Even though we sometimes limit prevention to 'preventive medicine' – what the doctor does to keep the patient healthy – it is still true that prevention is far more than screening individual patients and vaccinating them and giving them drugs to keep their blood pressure and cholesterol down. Perhaps another view from outside – this time of malaria in history – may remind us of the wider scope of prevention.

'Since the beginning of history, malaria has killed half the men, women, and children that have died on this planet.'[1] Really? I don't know how to come up with, or evaluate, a statistic like that but I do know that still today, malaria is one of the leading killers, killing 2–3 million people a year, which is nearly 5% of all deaths in the world. That's about the same as the number that die yearly from AIDS. Yet malaria is curable and AIDS is not, and 40–50 years ago the World Health Organization was seriously talking about eradicating malaria. What happened? A brief review of history is revealing.

Since antiquity, people have not only known about malaria, but have tried to control it. Hippocrates in ancient Greece (400 BC) recognized that people who lived near marshes were more likely to get fevers, which recurred daily, every other day or every third day, and that those people developed large spleens. At the same time in ancient Rome, swamps were being drained for agriculture and the region flourished. Neglect of those drainage schemes, and the consequent increase in swamps and malaria, may have contributed to the downfall of the Roman Empire. Malaria, in fact, is an Italian word, 'mal'aria' (bad air), reflecting the early belief that it was the bad air, or 'miasma,' of swamps which caused malaria.

In other words, people felt, malaria was an **environmental** disease and changing – or avoiding – the environment where it flourished prevented the disease. This concept is obviously still valid. European settlers in Africa and India sought higher, malaria-free areas to live and the boarding school my children attended in Kenya is located at 7500 feet on purpose, to avoid malaria, risk for the missionary children, since malaria is rarely transmitted at that altitude. Even before people knew anything about the biological cause of malaria, they had a pretty good idea about how to prevent it – or at least avoid it.

By the 17th century, people could not only avoid malaria, they could also cure it. Jesuit missionaries to South America found the local people using the bark of a tree to treat fever, and they brought some of it back to Europe, where malaria also flourished. This was quinine from the cinchona trees of the Andes, one of the earliest drugs to enter the modern pharmacopoeia and still the gold standard of malaria treatment.

The problem in the 17th century was that people had not yet – and would not for another 200 years – generally accept that malaria was a **microbial** disease, even though they were treating it as such. They used the 'Jesuit's bark' for treatment, but they also used bleeding and purging to restore the imbalances they felt were present. When Oliver Cromwell got fever in 1658, he wanted nothing to do with the Jesuit's bark because he saw it as related to the Catholic Church, and anyone dabbling in 'popery' was a traitor. He remained religiously pure, but he died of malaria.

By 1880, when Pasteur and Koch were in their heyday proving microbial causes of many diseases, the Frenchman Alphonse Laveran identified the *Plasmodium* parasite as the cause of malaria, and won a Nobel prize for his efforts. Now people knew what they were treating with quinine, and Robert Koch became an advocate of using quinine prophylaxis for prevention as well. Agricultural schemes in Europe and North America had already drained swamplands earlier in the century, but malaria was still endemic in southern Europe and throughout the tropics. Drainage was not possible everywhere; 'Treat the patient,' said Koch, 'not the mosquito.'[2]

His comments on the mosquito referred to the other major tack research was taking in the late 19th century. Patrick Manson, author of the first edition of *Manson's Tropical Diseases* (now in its 21st edition), felt that people got malaria by drinking swamp water. But when another Englishman, Ronald Ross, suggested that mosquitoes had something to do with malaria, Manson encouraged him to research this in India where Ross had been posted, and advised him by mail. Ross eventually demonstrated the complete vector cycle for bird malaria in 1898, having already found evidence of human malaria in *Anopheles* mosquitoes the year before. An Italian, Giovanni Grassi, actually demonstrated the complete vector–host cycle for human malaria, but Ross won the Nobel prize.

Now the world had an additional way to view malaria, as a **vector-borne** disease, and Ross himself became a crusader for mosquito control as the main way to prevent the disease. It was this vector control approach that William Gorgas used in 1908 to rid the Panama Canal zone of malaria and yellow fever. Twenty years earlier, these diseases had defeated the French in their attempt to dig the canal but with the diseases gone, the Americans completed the canal. Wilson and Soper of the Rockefeller Foundation used the same approach to stem a devastating Brazilian epidemic in 1938.

But these successes were just the beginning. With the development of DDT in the 1940s, the world had an effective tool to use with the vector approach. Spraying house walls with DDT killed mosquitoes and the effect lasted for months. The idea was that if DDT broke malaria transmission by killing infected mosquitoes and then people with malaria were treated (with the then new, highly effective chloroquine) to eliminate the human parasite reservoir, malaria in that region could be not just controlled but eradicated.

Eradicated. Done away with completely. This had never happened before, with any disease. But after World War II, America was on a high. It had won the war, then magnanimously helped to rebuild Europe and Japan. It would commit itself to putting a person on the moon by the end of the 1960s, and succeed. Technology in medicine was galloping forward and life in America seemed pretty good. So in the 1950s the World Health Organization, backed by American optimism and money ($3/4 billion between 1956 and 1969), committed itself to eradicate malaria from the world.

It was an interesting idea and it worked – in four European countries, five island countries, and Chile. It came close to succeeding in several other countries (India is an important example) but the program was not continued until the last parasite was gone and malaria came back, and with a vengeance. Eradication ultimately failed everywhere in the tropics except Africa, where it couldn't fail because it had hardly even gotten started.[3]

What happened? In analyzing the failure of malaria eradication, the World Health Organization realized that there was something wrong (they called it 'a wide and deep-seated error') with the distribution of basic health services world-wide. In 1978 their response, together with UNICEF, was to proclaim that by focusing our attention on primary healthcare, the world would have 'Health For All By The Year 2000.'

The resulting system of primary healthcare has merit, even though its accompanying slogan proved to be presumptuous. It seeks to involve community people in their own appropriate health system, combining basic treatments and preventive measures for the most common diseases. In addition, it is built on a model like the Chinese 'barefoot doctor' system, thereby reducing dependence on expensive, highly trained doctors as the first line of care in every village. The UN uses its technical resources not to deliver the care but to suggest which disease and environmental conditions would be the most efficient to focus on, and to suggest appropriate technologies to use.

It was clear early on, with this approach, that there were a few big deficiencies in the Third World: water, sanitation, and food. The diarrhea and malnutrition they caused were pivotal reasons for poor health, especially among children. Working on the problems of food and water, together with health education about sanitation and the use of oral rehydration for the early treatment of diarrhea, became the cornerstones of primary healthcare. Before long it became clear that respiratory disease in these under-nourished children was as potent a killer as diarrhea, and the UN developed suggestions and protocols for its management as well.

In other words, the UN was treating these diseases not just as environmental or microbial but as **recurrent, endemic, and inter-related** conditions that needed constant attention for their control, not their eradication. And for most of the first two decades of primary healthcare, malaria was not included as a specific focus. Eradication of this vector-borne disease had failed, but it was still viewed somehow differently from the other endemic diseases. It was almost as if the world community was embarrassed about their dramatic failure and in the coming years, instead of addressing malaria, they ignored it. Malaria, of course, did not go away.

In reality, malaria is not only an environmental disease, a microbial disease, and a vector-borne disease but it is also a recurrent, endemic disease, related to the other endemic diseases which contribute to poor health. This insight is, officially at least, quite new. In 1995 the USAID began its 'Africa Integrated Malaria Initiative' to emphasize that malaria deserves the same kind of attention that primary healthcare has given malnutrition, diarrhea, and pneumonia, and needs to be 'integrated' with them into primary healthcare. The Integrated Management of Childhood Illnesses (IMCI) program grows from the same assumption. Perhaps the embarrassment is over. But if it is, our problems with malaria prevention certainly aren't. If malaria is a recurrent endemic condition related to other recurrent endemic conditions, that makes it a **chronic** problem, pointing us back to the comments on chronic diseases a few chapters back. If the concept of taking medicine for the rest of one's life is foreign, so too will be the concept of doing anything repeatedly to prevent a disease, such as weekly chemoprophylaxis or seasonally treating a mosquito net with insecticide. Perhaps we haven't finished articulating paradigms for malaria control.

Now let us return to the diseases of the West. How can this brief guided tour through the history of malaria control help us to think about prevention and confront our own plagues?

Mainly this: how we as a profession – or as a whole society – view a disease makes a big difference in how we try to control it. Koch and Ross had access to the same research findings, but their approaches were very different. Koch wanted to treat the patient with quinine for prophylaxis or cure; Ross advocated instead control of the mosquito vector. The Ross approach led eventually to the attempts in the 1950s to eradicate malaria, which failed. The Koch emphasis resurged by default in the 1970s when malaria control was being ignored. By the 1990s, we were 'integrating' malaria into primary healthcare. The difference is not in the disease but in our approach.

There are some lessons for AIDS control. If we view AIDS mostly as a microbial disease (which it is), we will put money and effort into seeking a cure and a vaccine. If we view it as a sexually transmitted disease (which it also is), our focus will be on health education and, possibly, condom distribution. Can we also view it as a behavioral disease, the consequence of frequent unprotected sex with people likely to be infected? Or as a disease of poverty, as we heard Mbeki suggest in Chapter 8? If so, what are the implications for our preventive efforts? The easy response is that it is all of these, and needs a multi-pronged approach. But in our divided society, we have Ross camps and Koch camps, each seeking money for their cause. How do we decide which approach to take? Our current emphasis is on triple drug therapy and we are trying to export this to Africa, the very place malaria eradication didn't fail because lack of infrastructure meant it never even got started. Africa still lacks infrastructure and resistance to antiretrovirals is increasing. Will we some day view drug treatment of AIDS the way we now view malaria eradication?

Or a question closer to home: heart disease. If we view atherosclerosis as basically a biochemical abnormality, it makes sense to give drugs that lower the levels of serum lipids and blood pressure. If, on the other hand, we view atherosclerosis as a disease resulting from lifestyle, we will put our attention on diet and exercise counseling. If we step back further and view atherosclerosis as a disease of industrialization, we may consider advocating for less industry or advising our patients to move to places with no industry.

Again, we are likely to affirm that heart disease is all of these and that prevention requires biochemical, lifestyle, and even societal changes. But where do we physicians put most of our attention? And consequently, what is the message to our patients? We may affirm the necessity of change on many levels, but our training makes us most comfortable with biochemical adjustments. Even when we 'prescribe' exercise and diet, we are following the 'biomedical' model: how many minutes per day of aerobic exercise is helpful, how many calories from fat are dangerous. Our belief may be that diet and lifestyle are the most important but we likely spend more *time* with our patients talking about cholesterol and blood pressure levels.

What, then, is our responsibility in prevention? It is undoubtedly our task to diagnose – and yes, to diagnose early – and certainly to treat. Primary care physicians, the 'gate-keepers' for the entire system, should also be able to advise people on how to avoid coming through the gate. But we should not assume that gate-keepers are the core of prevention, especially when those preventive activities are rooted in our biomedical paradigm. Our contribution is part, but only part, of keeping people healthy.

Nevertheless, could we or should we be doing more? For those of us truly interested in health and prevention, is it possible to envision a doctor who truly coordinates all the preventive activities of our patients? Should we be satisfied with only the biomedical parts, with viewing disease only the way Koch did, and letting someone else be Ronald Ross?

Whether or not we want to, we physicians are likely to be limited to biomedical prevention and the reason brings us back once again to paradigms. If we try to engage in serious educational or nutritional counseling, we find ourselves stepping on the toes of health educators and nutritionists. If we enter seriously into true primary prevention, we become involved with community organizing, with advertising, with politics, and we have left clinical medicine altogether. There is no law keeping us from doing these things but they are seen in our society as the job of someone else. Our culture accepts specialization – demands it, even – and when we leave the box of clinical medicine for another box, we find ourselves being elbowed by people in that box. Specialization is a commonly agreed paradigm of how we function.

But most of us would not seriously think of spending much time in non-clinical activities, even if we enjoy them, because we don't get paid for them. Preventive activities take time and managed care tells us that we need to keep our encounters up. In other words, the financing system determines what is the best use of our time. Once again, we must function in a medical system based not on what is best for the public's health but what is best for the market – and these are rarely the same. Our financing paradigm can supersede our beliefs about health – and common sense.

However, the major point is not whether *physicians* spend time in preventive activities but, rather, whether or not prevention is being addressed by the medical system as a whole.[4] We have been struggling with malaria for centuries, alternating between dramatic success and tragic failure in our attempts to prevent the disease. Only now are we beginning to emerge from an embarrassing time of ignoring it. Physicians do have a task to perform in prevention, even if it is just the 'biomedical' part. The important thing to remember is that it is only a part.

CULTURE

CHAPTER FOURTEEN

Culture

Densu asked Damfo: 'Do we love something and not hate what goes against it?'
'You're right,' Damfo said. 'But for healing work love must be stronger than hate. Much stronger.'

Ayi Kwei Armah, *The Healers*

'Culture is a system of learned behaviors,'[1] behaviors determined by influences such as climate, natural resources, history, and religion. One of those influences is material resources – or lack of them. Consider this story I recorded after a visit to a rural clinic in Tanzania.

How often have I stood, sat or paced, waiting for the car to go? The anger begins even before the pre-arranged time to leave and by the time we are 10 minutes late, I am boiling inside. I need a Maalox; no, I need to find out why we haven't left yet. No, that never works; there's always a reason, an excuse. At least I should find someone to blame or better still, someone to yell at. Sometimes I do.

One morning we were going to Nyarero, six of us, and we were supposed to leave at 6 a.m. I arrived at 6, ready to begin pacing, to blame the driver for not preparing the car the day before, to wonder out loud where all the passengers were. But for some strange reason all six of us were there and by quarter past we were in the car driving out of the hospital parking lot.

I remarked with pleasure that we were leaving on time.

'Yes,' Dina laughed, 'I got here at five this morning.'

'Five?' I asked. 'Why so early?'

'Oh, when I got up I didn't know what time it was, so I came right here, and when I arrived the guard said it was only five.'

'You don't have any clocks in your house?'

'No.'

(Gulp)

I took a poll of those in the car: only three of us had any kind of clock or watch. The driver was not one.

Then Dina told me the rooster was her clock. She had two of them but had recently slaughtered one. 'You slaughtered your clock?' I asked. That brought laughter and then more chuckles that resurfaced for over 10 minutes.

It was the resource gap but with a new twist. The gap glared silently at me for my recurrent anger, and silenced me. There was the fleeting thought, 'Give them all a watch,' which I was answering even before I finished thinking it. The resource doesn't bridge the gap. People aren't late because they lack watches; they lack watches because they have a different sense of time. No, they lack watches because they lack money, but watches won't make people hoard time the way we hoard gold.

I didn't use any Maalox on that trip.

Visitors to rural and traditional cultures are often struck by the relaxed approach to time they encounter there. When those visitors are from the industrialized West and are either paying for their trip or trying to accomplish something, they find the local understanding of time frustrating and wasteful. The people they are visiting often find *them* rushed, rude, and impersonal. Yet neither approach to time, relaxed or rigid, is inherently better than the other. Each has advantages and disadvantages but neither is 'right.' That is the essence of culture: a way of doing things that the 'insiders' adopt unconsciously, without even realizing there is another way until they visit another culture.

But the story of the watches also underlines the complex relationship between culture and resources: do people have a relaxed view of time because they can't afford watches? Or do they not buy watches because they have a relaxed sense of time? More important than answering that question is realizing that the learned behaviors of a culture are intimately related to the availability of resources. More on this below.

Time is of course only one aspect of culture, only one place where cross-cultural relationship can lead to conflict. How readily people talk with strangers, whether or not they say 'Thank you', how often they bathe, which side of the street they drive on, whether they value independence and solitude or conformity and community – all these are the learned behaviors of culture. Clearly, then, how people respond to affliction is also culturally determined, as is the approach of healthcare providers to them. Yet as we saw with paradigms in Chapter 3, it is difficult to describe what everyone assumes, partly because there is usually no need to.

However, when people do cross cultural boundaries to work, as healthcare workers often do, the need to articulate cultural differences becomes very important. And as American society becomes more openly multicultural, all healthcare workers need to consider these differences, even if they never travel outside America.[2] In this chapter I want to look at three inter-related aspects of cross-cultural work: confronting the culture of the patients, the culture of medical staff, and the culture of the medical system itself.

The patients

When we enter another culture, we are often struck immediately by what is different from our own. And often, if we have chosen to enter that culture (rather than being forced to enter it), we like some of what we see; we feel 'they' do things better than 'we' do. This is usually a phase, lasting days to months. Eventually, however, we get tired of the difference or we begin to see the problems in the way they do things or we get frustrated that their way prevents us from doing our task. This is sometimes called 'culture shock' but it is usually a more gradual process than the term 'shock' suggests, and lasts longer. The following story illustrates how ubiquitous this experience is, this time looking at language rather than time.

We used to attend an annual East Africa retreat for missionaries and development workers from our organization, many with long-term experience working in other cultures. In previous years we had discussed development (and played volleyball) *ad nauseam*. One year the 'cutting edge' was 'relationships' (and still volleyball), and I was asked to co-lead a daily workshop on 'Relationship With Partners' – possibly because it was known that our relationship with our African partners was sometimes rocky.

On the third day we played this game: we were all supposed to be North American young married people living in a small North American town. We were unsatisfied with the traditional birthing arrangements in town (hospital and doctor dominant) and were meeting to discuss the building of a 'birthing center.' The rules of the game were intended to help us feel the realities of the cross-cultural situation we all lived in: 1) we would all sit in a circle; 2) anyone late needed to be welcomed by everyone, and have the rules explained by women; 3) women could only say five words at a time.

The meeting rapidly became uncomfortable. A few women tried to express feelings about why a birthing center was needed, talking in monotones, counting words. Soon the main emotion they were expressing was anger at being unable to say more than five words at once. Meanwhile the men tried to act normally, talking about square footage, cost, and the legal status of midwives. The sense was that since the women couldn't fully participate, the best route was for the men to move ahead and get the job done. No one tried to solve the communication problem and no one suggested that the men voluntarily restrict themselves to five words each to 'equalize' things.

The women's anger increased, until they finally all left to have a 'caucus' by themselves. While they were gone, the men tried to continue the discussion but they did wonder about sending a delegate to the women to hear and bring back their thoughts. It was only one suggestion, never acted on; the men had work to do.

Then the women ran back in with machine guns and gunned down all the men.

The discussions afterwards were even more revealing than the game. Annetta was angry at the rules, and at me for making them. Tim, a lawyer, wondered why the women didn't maximize their potential and try to find some way to communicate. Mark wondered why no one proposed that after every five words a woman said, someone would interject 'and . . .' or 'yes . . .' allowing her to go on.

It was not hard for anyone to link the experience of the game with our experience of dealing with African partners. Several people could appreciate that in the 'development game' the outsiders often dominate and the nationals become frustrated and angry. But Harold, who worked for an African organization, wondered if perhaps the outsiders were the ones with only five words in an African circle, and that the 'African game' leaves us outsiders frustrated and in the dark.

Either way, cultural patterns of communication can be a major barrier to health workers when they work cross-culturally. But the barriers are not insurmountable. Recognizing differences as cultural rather than moral is a first step. Respecting what is different is equally important. Being willing to temporarily put my culture aside, and act according to 'their' culture when I am working with 'them,' goes a long way to bridging the culture gaps. Even simply greeting people in their own language covers a multitude of sins.

But we do not need to 'go native' in order to work effectively in another culture. When William Stringfellow, a white theologian/lawyer, went to live in Harlem to practice law, he continued to have his shoes shined every day. One of the residents noticed this unusual behavior and commended him on it. Stringfellow reflected:

> In order . . . to be a person in Harlem, in order that my life and work there should have integrity, I had to be and to remain whoever I had become as a person before coming there. To be accepted by others, a man must first of all know himself and accept himself and be himself wherever he happens to be. In that way, others are also freed to be themselves. To come to Harlem involved, thus, no renunciation of my own past or of any part of it . . . What was necessary was just to be myself.[3]

The medical staff

If we travel to another culture for a short-term 'missions trip' or to meet an emergency, we often take our own support staff with us. We don't want to be a drain on the local community; we want to be self-sufficient, and mostly, we want to be efficient. We may be aware of the difficulties in crossing a culture and we try to short-cut them by being self-contained.

However, when we go to another culture for a longer time to work in healthcare, our co-workers – doctors, nurses, aids, clerks – will often be from the culture we are serving. Most of the time this is an advantage: they can interpret for us the responses of our patients and teach us some of the most intimate parts of the culture. They often become our closest friends. However, as the friendships develop, we can forget that they too are from the same culture and when cultural misunderstandings with these co-workers develop, they are particularly painful because we work so closely together. When we are in the 'honeymoon' phase of cultural adjustment and everything about the culture is wonderful, our co-workers are an added gift. But when the culture begins to irritate us, our co-workers can magnify that irritation.

That irritation, however, does not have to be a bad thing. When we first went to Africa to work in a refugee settlement in Sudan, we were told that our biggest conflict would be with our expatriate co-workers, and it was. In our second assignment, we got close enough to our Tanzanian co-workers to experience real conflict with them, and realized on some level that we were making progress. The progress continued: in a later assignment in Kenya, I had the following experience with my boss, Dr Lugaria.

Dr Lugaria and I tended to work quite differently. I liked septrin for childhood pneumonia, he liked amoxicillin. I was boisterous when I made rounds, he was very quiet. If I were in charge of something, I'd much prefer to delegate duties, even at the risk of the job not getting done. He knew that if he did something, it would get done – so he did it. It's probably good that he was the boss and I the employee.

Sometimes our different styles led to conflict. One time I made a decision on a patient I had been following after consulting with a surgeon; he saw the patient that evening, consulted with another surgeon, came to another decision, and changed my orders. More than once, on nights he was on call, he returned to the hospital at 10 or 11 after pursuing some administrative task, leaving us to cover on evenings we had hoped to be off.

Now I know that doctors everywhere are taught to form their own opinions and defend them, so conflict between doctors is not unusual. I also know that in African culture Dr Lugaria was not acting inappropriately. Africans have a more flexible view of time than Westerners, and a more hierarchical style of leadership. I may have been a Western doctor but I was working in an African hospital and the onus was on me to do things their way, not vice versa. Consequently, challenging Dr Lugaria would have been inappropriate. But I did challenge him a couple of times, asking him why he had changed my orders, and again why he was so late. Each time he knew I was upset but I doubt he saw these incidents as deserving the attention I was giving them. To me, he had trodden on my opinion and personal-time toes. To him, I was making mountains out of molehills. I left these run-ins delivered of my gripes but not very satisfied. He must have left them puzzled about why I was so riled.

Puzzled maybe, yet aware that there was a hitch in our relationship; aware that regardless of why, things weren't smooth between us. And aware, I later concluded, that it was up to him to begin the repair.

Our car had needed some bodywork done on it and he had recommended a man in his church whom he knew he could trust but whose shop was at least 45 minutes away. One afternoon after the car had been there for several weeks – and during the time that our latest run-in was still fresh in our minds – he suggested that we drive out to the shop to see how things were going. He had a few other stops to make on the way and of course, there was tea at his friend's shop and some purchases in Bungoma on the way back, so by the time the afternoon was over, we had spent five hours together, just he and I. We never mentioned the run-ins but we both knew that our relationship had been healed.

One reason to give special attention to the cross-cultural relationships with our staff is that we work so closely with them. They can be our teachers; they can, if we let them, heal us. But beyond this, our colleagues can be an important window to us into another way to practice 'our' Western, allopathic medicine. It is this third area, the medical system itself, which allows us to bring the outside view back home.

The medical system

When we work in America with people of other cultures, we may have all of the experiences noted above but we are still trying to practice medicine as we were taught it in the USA. But when we go to a Third World country to work, we need to adjust not only to the people we are working with but also to the entire medical system. This may lead us into some of the same experiences we have in confronting any other aspect of the culture – with one difference: we are less likely to have an initial feeling that everything is wonderful. The overall culture may have ancient roots and may preserve wisdom from the past but the culture (i.e. learned behaviors) of the medical system has developed much more recently. It will likely be a blend of traditional and Western understandings of healing, both struggling in a resource-poor environment.

Consequently, our initial impression of awe is not because everything is so wonderful but rather because everything is so poor. We may be shocked to see open wards with two or three people in a bed, IVs hanging from wires wrapped around the rafters, and a pervasive smell of urine. We get used to this but it is much more difficult to get used to what we see as apathy, inefficiency, and stubbornness in the clinic or hospital staff. No one hurries for emergencies, no one seems to care when people are hurting, no one wants to change the way they've always done things. We're in culture shock but we don't recognize it; it just seems to us that people don't know how to practice medicine.

I recorded the story of my own cross-cultural journey in Chapter 10, Healing. That journey involved not only adjusting to medicine in African culture (the step after culture shock) but also coming home and seeing the medical system I was trained in with new eyes, with a view from outside. I want to return to that journey now to articulate in more detail some of the differences between the Western allopathic medicine I was trained in and the way that same medicine is practiced in a culture with much more limited resources. There is of course benefit in looking at other paradigms of healing to see what they can teach us, and we will do this in the next chapter. But the focus here is on our own Western medical paradigm as described in Chapter 3, seen through the eyes of a different *culture*.

The fulcrum of Western allopathic medicine is diagnosis. Our medicines and surgeries are disease specific and we employ them only when we have a pretty good idea (or know = *gnosis*, part of *diagnosis*) what we are treating. Consequently we use the highest level people in our system, doctors, for diagnosis. Doctors can now delegate this task to nurse practitioners and physician's assistants but are still legally responsible. Most medicines are available only by prescription – of the doctor.

This system makes sense until we consider that in any community, the largest disease burden will consist of only a few diagnoses. Most sick children in tropical Africa will have malaria or pneumonia or diarrhea; most sick children in the USA will have common colds or ear infections. A large percentage of chronically ill adults on an American Indian reservation will have diabetes or hypertension. Many of these conditions are not difficult to diagnose or treat but we still rely primarily on doctors for all diagnosis and treatment. Rural Africa, not having enough doctors to be involved with every diagnosis, relies primarily on nurses for outpatient diagnosis and treatment. The fulcrum is not fine-tuned diagnosis but presumptive diagnosis to allow for readily available mass treatment. And it works. Our 'obsession' with a highly accurate, fine-tuned diagnosis for every patient is cultural, not scientific.

This fine-tuning in all of our work is a characteristic of Western medicine. We have extremely accurate laboratory and imaging studies and we use the most accurate (and most expensive) tests, even if the results will make little or no difference to the patient's health. This need to know exactly what is going on comes from our belief that the more information we have, the better off we are. This is cultural belief: we want to miss nothing.

But now it's not only physicians who don't want to miss anything; our patients want us to find everything, and so do their lawyers. Even if we feel that further information will not help our patient, we are afraid to not get it. We are all part of a culture that honors laboratory tests more than clinical judgment, a culture that assumes that looking harder will uncover all sources of present or future disease. The belief that all disease can be measured this way is a cultural belief. While wanting to know (*diagnosis*) is not cultural, wanting to know *everything* is.

Possibly the most extreme form of this wanting to know and measure everything is what Ivan Illich called 'the medicalization of life.'[4] Medicalization is describing in medical terms and treating as disease parts of our lives that aren't true illnesses: birth, pregnancy, menopause, old age, baldness, small breasts, grey hair, crooked teeth, impotence, motion sickness, anxiety, loneliness. Medicine of course may have a role in each of these situations. The problem is not in offering a hospital birth for a mother with a high-risk pregnancy, or an antihistamine for motion sickness, or braces for a child with crooked teeth. The problem is that the people who choose to get 'treatment' for these situations go to the same place as those with diseases; they, and the medical system, treat these stages or variants as diseases. Eventually we all consider them as diseases and assume everyone should get 'treatment,' even those who don't want it. The most recent addition to this list is the medicalization of risk, discussed in Chapter 12, Prevention – 1.

Third World medicine cannot afford to medicalize all of life, fortunately. But more than this, most Third World cultures don't have the same obsession with measuring and fine-tuning and knowing everything and predicting that we do. These cultural traits have all become part of our medical system and it takes a view from outside to see that they are *cultural* traits, not inherent to the practice of good allopathic Western medicine.

CHAPTER FIFTEEN

Learning

The learner [wishing to be a healer] avoids going to any place where men go to seek power over other men.

Ayi Kwei Armah, *The Healers*

The underlying theme of this whole book is that looking at our Western health-care system with an 'outside' view can give us a deeper understanding of our own strengths and weaknesses. Besides seeing our own culture of medicine more clearly, another way we can learn from this outside view is to examine specifically how other cultures carry out healthcare, and consider which parts we can adopt. This is a new approach for some involved in international health. Until the last decade, 'international health' implied the study of and involvement in Third World countries by European and North American health professionals, in order to help the poor in those Third World countries. The subject matter was mostly 'tropical medicine'; the motivations were some combination of altruism and adventure. Even the United Nations 'Health for All' initiatives beginning in the 1970s, to be accomplished by a new understanding of primary healthcare, were focused on the Third World, though admittedly with increasing respect for Third World solutions. The assumptions were still that the Third World was 'in need' and that countries less 'in need' could help fill that need.[1,2]

Recently, however, there has been an increasing awareness that international health is much more than this. While the predominant perception of international health is still that of 'us helping them,' some US physicians experienced in international health have been asking how this experience could be turned back to help us.[3] In 1993, the National Council for International Health (now called Global Health Council) published *Global Learning For Health*, a book-length collection of experiences and reflections on how international perspective and experience can help so-called developed countries address their own health problems. The center of gravity was shifting. By 1999, Drs Cal Wilson and Ron Pust could propose a comprehensive definition for international health that showed how much thinking had changed from the assumption that international health was just 'exporting doctors to a world in need.'

> The discipline of international health is directed toward helping enhance health in diverse populations and cultural contexts, encompassing the multiple environmental, socio-cultural, political, and biologic factors involved. This discipline is best pursued by the bilateral exchange of knowledge and perspectives between more-developed and less-developed areas of the world.[4]

This is in some ways new territory, for international health at least. Only a decade ago international health was only what 'we' did for 'them.' Its academic centers were in the West, its 'laboratories' in the tropics. The standards were ours, the needs theirs.[5] Wilson and Pust's assumptions are radically different. They say that the focus is the health of everyone, not just people in the Third World. They recognize the laboratories to be wherever there are 'diverse populations and cultural contexts' and their academic centers are based in 'bilateral exchanges of knowledge and perspectives,' not Western assumptions.

Their definition, in other words, is about 'bringing international health back home,' a phrase Russell Morgan used in his introductory essay to *Global Learning for Health*.

Given, then, that international health is becoming truly inter-national, it may be appropriate to look more closely at how we can relate and learn from each other. There are two conflicting images, or paradigms, or understandings of how different peoples in the world relate to each other today. There is, on the one hand, 'globalization' and on the other, 'ethnicity.'

Globalization says 'the world is shrinking' so we're all part of the same 'global village.' Modern communication helps us to keep up with what's going on in different parts of that village. We have different histories and cultures but we are no longer isolated from each other. Though our problems may differ, my problem impacts on your problem, and my solution has fallout for your problem and for your solution. This paradigm says, 'Let's define the problem together, and identify the common thread. Let's work together on solutions we can both use.'

Ethnicity says we are more different than we are similar, and that because my history, my climate, and my culture are different from yours, so is my village. In fact, since modern communication is beginning to blur the differences between me and you, I must struggle to maintain my identity. We may have similar problems but the solution developed in your village may not work at all in mine. This paradigm of diversity does not ignore global problems, though; it says rather, 'Let me work on my problem within my culture, then let me share my story with you. I want to hear your story, too. But I'm the one that needs to apply your story to my village, just as you need to decide what to do with my story in your village.'

Globalization is often seen by the global intelligentsia as the inevitable way to future progress, supported by computer networks and based on research done in a scientific language understood world-wide. This intelligentsia sees the diversity rooted in ethnicity as enriching, but an impediment to progress when it is taken too seriously. In the extreme, globalization is seen as progressive, ethnicity regressive; globalization as leading to peace, ethnicity to war. Globalization claims the international 'moral high ground' as it tries to be inclusive and sees ethnicity as competitive and exclusive.

Indeed, who can deny that most wars today, especially in Africa, Eastern Europe and the former Soviet empire, and the Middle East, have ethnic roots? Case proven?

Not exactly. Ethnicity can be a problem when carried to extremes. But individual cultures hold and protect a great spectrum of indigenous wisdom, wisdom which can be diluted when passed through a global sieve. The full value of ethnic wisdom cannot be found in a global distillation of it. Globalization may appear to give ethnicity a voice but it does so on its own terms: 'least common denominator' terms. Ethnicities may see a threat in globalized homogeneity and respond by trying to politicize their culture (and wisdom) and defend it violently – or withdraw and hide. Yet without globalization, ethnicity cannot effectively offer its wisdom to the rest of the world. It is not easy to tap that great indigenous wisdom.

The importance of these paradigms for international health is this: as the discipline of international health increasingly becomes an exchange of ideas and experiences meant to benefit the health of *all* of us, it becomes more and more important to consider how we relate to each other and how we learn from each other. Do we all sit together at some sort of non-ethnic global table and offer our ethnic flavorings to a world stew? Or do we need to visit each other's huts and palaces in order to really know what local food is like?

In the new globalized international health, it appears that we begin with the non-ethnic global table. We develop recipes there, try them out in some huts and then come back to the table to work on the cookbook. It's a globalization paradigm; the rules are not ethnic (neither 'ours' nor 'theirs') but 'international.' It is an efficient, non-biased structure designed to facilitate the exchange of ideas – the ideas of those who make it to the table.

A couple of examples from *Global Learning for Health* will illustrate. There is a chapter there entitled 'Evolution of the La Leche League Mother-to-Mother Support: From the Suburbs of Illinois to Peri-Urban Communities in Central America and Back to the United States.' The title tells the story: an American idea was transformed by its immersion in the Third World and when it came back home, it was richer.

H. Jack Geiger's personal history of the US community health center movement is equally illustrative.[6] He makes it clear that the ideas behind the first US neighborhood health centers in 1965 were rooted in the experience of Sidney and Emily Kark in South Africa experimenting with community-oriented primary care there in the 1940s. They, La Leche, and many other authors in the volume explicitly acknowledge their debt to ideas developed in the Third World.

This is real international learning – of the globalization type. Community-oriented primary care may not be a particularly Western idea but there is nothing distinctly African about it either. It comes from the global table and so is intended for the whole globe. Because there is nothing 'ethnic' about it, it should be unwelcome nowhere. Therein lies its potential usefulness.

But this is only one kind of learning. There is other wisdom based in the ethnicity of a people, and sometimes that wisdom can enhance the health of all humankind. In the 17th century, for example, Jesuit missionaries in South America learned from the indigenous people that a certain tree bark was a good treatment for malaria. That tree bark contained quinine, which is still the 'gold standard' for malaria treatment.

Many traditional peoples have long had local 'bone-setters' who do an excellent job of treating some closed fractures. Are their methods applicable today? *Clinical Orthopaedics and Related Research* thinks so, and not long ago republished a classic 1963 article acknowledging the debt.[7] How many other drugs and techniques are buried within local cultures that never make it to the global table?

And beyond clinical medicine, do indigenous groups possess other wisdom that can benefit mankind's health? A review of several studies on the prognosis of schizophrenia concluded that 'the outcome of schizophrenia in developing countries is generally more favorable.'[8] Why? Is there anything that the 'developed' world can learn from this? But more importantly, is there a way to bring this kind of question to the global table?

To summarize: international health has been evolving in the last decade from 'exporting doctors to a world in need' to a bilateral collaborative exchange of knowledge directed toward enhancing the health of humankind. The ways in which we learn from each other in this collaborative exchange are based either in a set of common assumptions about how we approach the task (called here 'globalization') or in a recognition of our separate and unique contributions (which I've called 'ethnicity'). Despite their apparent antagonism, both paradigms inform international communication and each has an important role. However, most people in the academic community find globalization a more comfortable paradigm in which to work. Consequently indigenous wisdom may well remain 'undiscovered' and thus unavailable for the health of humankind.

As international health continues to ask the larger questions about how the study of health in diverse populations and cultural contexts can enhance the health of all humankind, it is important to be explicit about how we ask the questions. There is certainly a role for looking at programs and systems developed at the global table and often put in place first in the Third World. This is the predominant paradigm behind the learnings in *Global Learning for Health*. But there is also a need to look within the 'diverse populations and cultural contexts' themselves for wisdom that may yet nourish all of us at the global table.

CHAPTER SIXTEEN

Poverty

I do not see us blindly fearing power. We healers do not fear power. We avoid power deliberately, as long as that power is manipulative power. There is a kind of power we would all embrace and help create. It is the same power we use in our work: the power of inspiration . . . But that kind of power . . . can never be created with manipulators. If we healers allow the speedy results of manipulation to attract us, we shall destroy ourselves and more than ourselves, our vocation.

Ayi Kwei Armah, *The Healers*

'The poor,' Jesus said, 'you have with you always.' It's a great line, not least because history seems to have proven it true. Some of us hide behind that simple statement as an excuse to do nothing for poor people. Others carry it on a banner to incite action on their behalf. Both reduce it to a truism, and both miss the point of why Jesus said it.

He was, it turns out, making a home visit to a man with leprosy shortly before Passover one year. He had already told his friends he expected to be killed soon, but most of them didn't understand what he meant. However, his friend Mary, Lazarus and Martha's sister, caught on better than the rest and after dinner, she poured some very expensive perfume on him, symbolically preparing his body for burial.

It was then that the discussion of poverty and the welfare system came up. 'Bad move,' several of them said, thinking of their budget. 'Very bad,' said Judas, the accountant. 'If this Disciples Club you've set up means anything,' they reasoned, 'it's that we're supposed to somehow help the poor. Now we were *this* close to getting a whole year's wages in the Fund, and this woman blew it on *perfume*. Then she dumped it all out at once!'

'You missed the point. Again,' said Jesus. 'There are two matters at stake here: worship and work, and the first undergirds the second. You've got the rest of your lives to work doing good for the poor – because, you know, they will always be with you – but, like I told you, I won't. Don't worry about the Fund; *be* the Fund yourselves. Now it's time to come here and say goodbye, kind of like Mary did.'

'Besides,' he might have added, 'you won't find the poor out there just now. They're in here with me, saying goodbye.'

Jesus' statement about poverty was an aside to his comments about worship. But it was an aside that implied ongoing work on behalf of the poor, at least for his followers. We don't have to be followers of Jesus, though, to learn something from this story. There are several points relevant to healthcare among poor people.

First is the whole matter of trying to get rid of poverty itself. We know that an ounce of prevention is worth a pound of cure and it's tempting to apply the same principle to poverty. Primary healthcare world-wide has tried to do this over the last two decades, as have various brands of socialism and communism over the last century. But many among us have been skeptical that eradication of poverty is possible, and with the recent international collapse of communism, there is a strong temptation to say, 'Naa, naa, I told you so. The poor you have with you always.'

Yes, and that statement was originally connected with the assumption that 'whenever you will, you can do good to them.' Just because we can't cure a cancer doesn't keep us from giving palliative chemotherapy. Should our inability to eradicate poverty keep us from caring for poor people? We can cut out some cancers and we can eliminate some conditions that produce poverty. If we try to hide behind Jesus' maxim in order to defend our inactivity, it backfires on us.

On the other hand, we have already seen what Jesus did with the activists: he showed them a case of blatant waste and said it wasn't. His problem was not with their activity on behalf of the poor but with their balance between work and worship. Yet beyond this confusion, there is the matter of the Fund we set up, the system that we put in place to help the poor. Judas the treasurer, we are told, was a thief; his concern for the preservation of the Fund was so that he could continue to dip into it. Any big fund, like welfare or Medicaid, is subject to abuse from either end, Fund managers as well as recipients. Jesus was not committed to protecting the Fund but he also does not allow potential Fund-bashers off the hook. The poor are always there, he said, to help.

We may agree that we are stuck with poverty, and we may even agree that the virtuous thing is to try somehow to help some poor people. But now things get complicated. Jesus had no statisticians to deal with and no insurance companies. His healing was very 'low tech', his costs were not spiraling – financial costs, that is. Our healthcare is far more complicated and so is our poverty. How do religious or ethical 'oughts' fit in a medical care system controlled by managed care priorities and technological imperatives? Besides, isn't that what the Health Department and federally funded clinics are for?

Yes, poverty is complicated and yes, there are systems set up to care for poor people – although those systems are more tentative than they seem, increasingly vulnerable in a market-dominated economy. 'Too bad,' some physicians say, 'that's not my problem.' But other physicians hold on to an ethic, possibly an echo of some assumptions Jesus made, and say, 'If we each did our part, it wouldn't be so bad.' Few of us relish the prospect of caring for poor people; it is, at best, an unpleasant responsibility that won't seem so bad if we would just all share it.

There is, however, another way to look at this business of treating poor people. Our assumption has been that if we are to care for poor people, it is because they need us. Could it be that the opposite is also true, that we need them? David Hilfiker suggests exactly this in an article,[1] to which I will return shortly. But since needing poor people may be a new concept to you, and can be felt more than explained, I would like to illustrate it with several stories. And since you may be tempted to appreciate from a distance – and dismiss – stories from Africa, I will use stories of American poor people.

It was never clear to me what Harold's chief complaint was. He fit fairly well in the disabled-from-his-nerves-and-back category but when he came for a visit, I wasn't sure why he was there that day, nor what he wanted from me. His chief complaint seemed to be to complain. He would sit with his hands on his knees, head downcast, and speak slowly of his pain and his temper. There would be a pause, and I would make a suggestion or concluding remark, but Harold was never quite finished. He seemed to not want to be there, yet was reluctant to leave.

Early on I had shared with him the wisdom of the pain–depression–pain cycle. He obliged me by attending a few counseling sessions and taking some antidepressants, neither of which affected him. He similarly eluded my attempts to nail down the exact organic nature of his problem: he either didn't go for referral visits or didn't return for follow-up.

He eventually realized the futility of visiting me, I suppose, and stopped coming for over a year. Then he returned periodically, usually at his wife's insistence, with the same slow speech, same set of complaints, same reluctance to leave.

Boots was the neighborhood sot, and lived alone near Harold. A couple of years previously his house had burned down ('faulty wiring') and after a few months in a trailer out of town with his son, he moved back to the neighborhood and into a shack built on the site of his burned home.

I first met Boots shortly before Thanksgiving when he had a hunting accident and put a bullet through his toe. Four hours after the accident, which happened at home, he called the Health Department asking only for a tetanus shot, and the public health nurse suggested he also see me. He explained that he had had one beer that morning to ease the pain and needed something stronger. I devised a plan for dressing changes, antibiotics, and pain pills, none of which he followed through on except the pain pills. I found him a few days later, got him the antibiotics, changed the dressing, and arranged for visiting nurses to see him daily. He eluded them after a few visits and stopped his antibiotics. He became 'lost to follow-up.'

Linda, Harold's wife, was a faithful patient. She had to be: she had severe asthma, with frequent attacks brought on by infection, Harold, and who knows what else. Shortly after Boots' accident, she told me her opinion: that Boots had intentionally shot himself to get pity from the neighbors and help splitting his wood.

Then, almost disgusted, she told me of Harold's mercy. Harold would drag Boots out of a ditch when he'd lain there day and night drunk, and Harold would sit talking for hours with Boots, encouraging sobriety. Harold's 'nerves got all tore up' when Boots got hurt or sick. After the house burned and Boots came back to the neighborhood, Harold let Boots stay in his shed, until Linda put a stop to that. So Harold, disabled, merciful Harold, got Boots to use his VA check one month for used lumber, and Harold built him his shack.[2]

Harold did far more for Boots than I ever did. My final act of mercy was, as medical examiner one hot summer day, to pronounce Boots' maggot-ridden body dead. I was a medical technician for Boots; any healing influence he felt came from Harold.

But poor people don't only help us to heal others. Sometimes we are the ones in need of healing. At the end of Hilfiker's article he tells this story.

Like many others in the city of Washington, John Williamson, 43, also known as PeeWee, had not had a home for almost a year when he was finally brought to the hospital for treatment. [He had pneumonia and AIDS. After discharge he was too weak to live on the streets and so was referred to Joseph's House, a home and community for formerly homeless men with AIDS, directed by Hilfiker.]

As far as we could determine, PeeWee had never used IV drugs himself but he had been a hustler all his life, living by his wits within the violence of the Washington streets. His stock answer to any of the other men who angered him, which he continued to repeat long after he'd withered to less than 90 pounds, was 'I'll kick the crap out of anyone who messes with me.' But PeeWee was also brutally honest and intensely loyal; he was able to recognize when he'd been wrong and knew how to apologize with sincerity.

At one of our community meetings a month or so after PeeWee arrived, another resident began complaining that 'someone' was talking disrespectfully to 'the staff.' Immediately PeeWee spoke up. 'I'll take that beef!' he said. 'You don't need to talk about 'someone' talking disrespectfully. That was me, and

I cursed Dixcy out. But I see that you all don't do that here. I was wrong and I apologize.' And PeeWee turned to Dixcy and said it again, straight to her face, 'I'm sorry, Dixcy. I shouldn't have said that, and it won't happen again.' It didn't . . .

Once he had accepted us as his family, he became a leader in the house. His death after nearly two years with us left a gaping hole in our community.

From one point of view, PeeWee epitomized everything that was wrong with the inner city. He was uneducated and illiterate; he'd lived by violence and by crime and rarely had a straight job. He'd gotten AIDS and found himself on the streets, abandoned by family and society. Yet he was able to become a cornerstone of our community because of his intelligence, forthrightness and honesty. He became my seventeen-year-old daughter's 'protector,' and when she left for Minnesota for college, he quite seriously told her that if anyone bothered her, she should call him and he would call friends in Minneapolis who would 'take care of it.'

When we as middle-class, affluent, relatively healthy caregivers place ourselves alongside people whose wounds are more obvious than our own, we are offered a mystery, a unique opportunity for healing.

I've suffered for years from clinical depression. I've done everything I know to do. I've prayed and been prayed for, taken medications of various stripes, done prolonged intensive psychotherapy with a Christian therapist, taken spiritual direction, practiced intense aerobic exercise, taken sabbaticals, meditated – you name it. It appears that my depression will never be healed; it will always be there crouched just beneath the surface, sometimes leaping out to overwhelm me.

Three years ago the depression started breaking through again and it became particularly agonizing. I intensified my prayer; I visited my psychiatrist and adjusted medications; I continued my therapy; I cut back on my work schedule. Nothing worked. Just before Christmas the intensity mounted and for the first time in my life I became dysfunctional. That scared me. I stopped work at my clinic but was still living at Joseph's House. The pressure of trying to be present to the men in the face of my depression, however, was too much.

I had from time to time shared in our community meetings about my depression but always with a certain clinical detachment that left me pretty much in control. This time there was no illusion of control. I talked about the acuteness of my depression – which, of course, was no surprise to the men since they'd been watching me like hawks. I talked about my fear of the chaos. I told them I would not be able to respond to them either as a doctor or as a person of responsibility in the house.

I stopped talking and sank back into myself, not knowing what to expect. Right away, PeeWee spoke up. 'That's cool, Doc. We been noticin' somethin' wrong. You just take as much time as you need. We'll still be here for you.' And over the next few minutes each of the men responded. I can't remember all their words but the feelings were the same. There was no overreaction, no soulful looks of deep understanding or pity, no embarrassment for me, no offers of help. Just simple acknowledgment that I was going through a rough time and that they would be there for me. One of the men said he'd pray for me.

There was no sudden cure to my depression, no flash of insight, but the healing to my soul was incalculable. I had acknowledged my utter brokenness and they weren't frightened by it, embarrassed by it, disgusted with it or eager to cure it. Just, 'That's cool, Doc. We'll be here for you.'

In our society, of course, we ghettoize these men and their brothers and sisters. They're the 'dope addicts,' the welfare queens, the criminals, the violent. We push them out of our sight because we are afraid of our own darkness, unwilling to look at our own vulnerability and brokenness. They become the repositories of all that fearfulness, hopelessness, valuelessness, meaninglessness that we cannot face in ourselves.

PeeWee, if you can believe his story – which I do – had been responsible for the deaths of several people in the violent drug world he'd inhabited for so many years before coming to Joseph's House. He was one of those we so fear when we think of the inner city. He was no stranger to his own brokenness. What he offered me was unpitying acknowledgment of my vulnerability and the awareness that some things will never be healed.

Part of the mystery is that the love and acceptance the men offered allowed me, over the next days and weeks, to become more aware of my depression as a certain kind of gift, as an entrance into the world of those I care for: I can no longer ignore my own brokenness and so am able to accept theirs without judgment. When they talk to me about their suffering – whether they know about my depression or not – they are aware that at some level I know what they are talking about.

It is a great gift.

Gifts like this may not be as rare as they seem. When I started looking for the gifts I'd received in my work with poor people, I found many, some as far back as my internship. And, as with David Hilfiker's story, they came to me most significantly when I needed them. This story is about . . . well, I forget his name but I'll give him one because he has always been more than a 'case' to me.

Albert was in his sixties, bald, black, and a barber. He had heart disease with major rhythm problems, meaning he felt OK most of the time, but we knew the extra beats in his heart could set off a dangerous and fatal arrhythmia at any time. Because of this we were giving him high doses of powerful drugs that were themselves dangerous.

One day the arrhythmia caused his heart to stop and we called a Code Blue to resuscitate him. It was successful but he still had the rhythm problem and we needed to adjust his medication. My resident suggested I restart him on the same high dose of the medicine we had used, beginning the next morning. I wrote the order but I forgot to write 'beginning in the morning.'

The next morning Albert had the arrhythmia again and stopped breathing again. We were nearby and so were able to insert a tube into his windpipe and breathe for him by squeezing the breathing bag. We also performed external cardiac massage which successfully kept his blood circulating. For 90 minutes interns took turns pumping on his chest while I squeezed the bag and the residents tried every way they could to give medications to regulate his heart. By this time it was clear to me that the reason for this tragedy was not his own heart problem but the toxicity of the medication that we were giving him; excess medicine that he had gotten throughout the night because I had neglected to write the order properly.

In other words, I knew he was dying now not from his disease but from his treatment that I had mistakenly given him. After 90 minutes he was still alive – he'd twist his head and grimace. But after 90 minutes we had been completely unsuccessful in making his heart beat on its own. We decided to stop trying; I stopped 'bagging' him and he died. We all felt bad but I felt more than bad; I felt guilty. Something that I had done (or not done or done wrong – it amounted to the same thing) had caused Albert's death. In other words, I had unwittingly killed him.

Is that melodramatic? I don't know. I have never intended to take anyone's life but several times since then I have made mistakes that resulted in someone's death, and I always feel like the bottom has fallen out. That was the first time and the bottom did fall out. I stood on the ward, surrounded by patients and doctors, the paint on the MD after my name still wet, and I started crying. Not just tears staining my face: I was sobbing. And one of the attendants came up to me and put her arm around my shoulder.

But the story does not end there. A day or two later, Albert's wife came back to the hospital. When I heard she was around, I made it a point to be somewhere else; I couldn't face her. When I returned to the ward, I found that she had brought Albert's penknife as a gift for me.

For a long time I didn't know what to do with this story. I told the first part freely – possibly to try to expiate my guilt, to atone – but I didn't understand the part about the penknife. I was embarrassed by it. I found it easier to admit my mistake than to accept a gift I didn't deserve. I stuffed the penknife in my pocket, took it home and eventually lost it.

But the great gift, which I eventually recovered, was not the penknife. It wasn't even the gratitude the knife represents; Albert's wife probably never knew I made a mistake. The great gift was this: Albert's wife acted toward me in a way consistent with her culture, while I was treating myself according to my culture. It took me many years to recognize that my culture needed to be complemented by hers. Simply being who she was – while I was being who I was – was a gift. Perhaps it took living in Albert's ancestral homeland to make sense out of it; I don't know. But now the story resonates with much that has since happened to me.

Everyone who treats poor people gets penknives from patients, but many of us don't know what to do with them. Sometimes we don't even know we've been given a gift. We are here to serve, to give, and when someone tries to wash our feet, to share something very dear, to *teach* us, we don't get it. Maybe that's because we want to change things, not be changed. That's OK: things need changing. But if we lose the penknives, as I did, we lose something very precious.

David Hilfiker goes a step further. At the end of his story I just related, he asks, 'Is it then necessary that each of us move into the ghetto, spend full time in working with the poor?' He immediately answers, 'Of course not.' But he adds this:

> I'd like to suggest, however, that in our day and time, each of us must be in face-to-face contact with the poor at least two hours a week if we are to understand our society and ourselves. It might be volunteer work at a downtown shelter. It may be taking on several poor patients in our suburban practice. It may be attendance at a church in a poor neighborhood. It may mean tutoring kids once a week. Whatever it is, when we begin to see the world from the point of view of the poor, our world will change and the nature of reality will be clearer. To keep our vision clear, we need the poor.

Hilfiker is saying that all of us need a view from outside, which is what this book has been about. He is not suggesting that we treat poor people because they need us but because we need them, that 'the nature of reality will be clearer.' There is no promise that it will be fun, no suggestion that it is easy. There is only the assertion that 'to keep our vision clear, we need the poor.'

And, if we can hold on to them, the possibility of a pocketful of penknives.

Endnotes

Chapter One Introduction

1 See, for example, Himmelstein D, Woolhandler S, Hellander I (2001) *Bleeding The Patient: the consequences of corporate healthcare* (Common Courage Press).

Chapter Two Health

1 I based my studies on the work Maurice King reported in the second chapter of his *Medical Care in Developing Countries* (Oxford University Press, 1966).

2 See the discussion of the role of transportation in late 19th- and early 20th-century American medicine in *The Social Transformation of American Medicine* by Paul Starr (Basic Books, 1982), pp. 65–71.

3 This is not a new insight. In 1959, Rene Dubos wrote, concerning health in Western Europe and North America in the 19th century, that 'improvement clearly began long before the modern era in medicine was ushered in by the germ theory of disease' and 'by the time laboratory medicine came effectively into the picture the job had been carried far toward completion by the humanitarians and social reformers . . .' (*The Mirage of Health*, Harper and Row, 1959, pp. 21 and 23).

4 The thesis of Thomas McKeown's *The Role of Medicine: dream, mirage or nemesis?* (Princeton University Press, 1979) is that 'medicine is not vitally concerned with the major determinants of health' (p. 123).

5 *Ibid.*, pp. 138–9. McKeown makes a difference between 'standard of care (how well we do what we do)' and 'effectiveness of care (whether what we do is worth doing)'. He suggests that Americans are more concerned with standard of care, while the British focus more on effectiveness.

Chapter 3 Paradigms

1 From Chapter 1 of Thorn GW (1977) *Harrison's Principles of Internal Medicine*, 8th edn, McGraw Hill, New York.

2 *Webster's New World Dictionary of the American Language*, college edition, 1964.

3 Starr P (1982) *The Social Transformation of American Medicine*. Basic Books, p. 100.

4 Op. cit., *Webster's New World Dictionary.*

5 Janzen JM (1980) *The Development of Health.* Development Monograph Series #8. Mennonite Central Committee, p. 14.

6 Janzen, *ibid.*, p. 9. Louise Lander, in *Defective Medicine: risk, anger, and the malpractice crisis* (Farrar, Straus, and Giroux, 1978), says the same thing: 'The germ theory and its historic predecessors, which have viewed disease as an *attack* from outside . . . have long competed for acceptance with a conception of illness as an ecological *disequilibrium* within . . .' (my emphasis), p. 79.

7 Janzen, *op. cit.*, pp. 11–14.

8 Lander (*op. cit.*, p. 79), in fact, refers to 'the triumph of the germ theory . . .'

9 Some Family Physicians accept the 'bio-psychosocial' paradigm of disease, rather than the more narrow 'biomedical.' It is a difficult stance to maintain: many teachers and most colleagues of Family Physicians function according to the 'biomedical' paradigm.

Chapter 4 Hubris

1 These quotes, and all of the Greek stories I've used, are from Edith Hamilton's 1940 *Mythology.* A Mentor book from New American Library, Times Mirror, New York.

2 Krauthammer C (1996) A lack of maternal instinct. *Guardian Weekly*, **154**(22).

3 Pantheon, 1976.

4 All quotes from *ibid.*, pp. 32–4, 41 and 127.

5 *Ibid.*, p. 270.

6 Illich I (1995) Pathogenesis, immunity, and the quality of public health. *Qual Health Res.* 5(1): 7. Illich I (1990) Health as one's own responsibility – no, thank you!, based on a speech given in Hannover, Germany, Sept 14, available at http://www.davidtinapple.com/Illich/

7 A less sensational way to say the same thing refers to 'the paradox of health.' Despite increasing technology and even measurable improvements in health status, 'people now report higher rates of disability, symptoms, and general dissatisfaction with their health' (Barsky A (1988) The paradox of health. *NEJM.* 318(7): 414–18).

Chapter 5 Ethics

1 From articles in the *Guardian Weekly* (2000) **163**(10): 9, and **163**(12): 10, 13.

2 Morris S (2000) 'Unlawful killing' dilemma in Siamese twin case. *The Guardian Weekly.* 163(12): 10.

3 It is odd when the oldest fetal age of legal abortion approaches, and even passes, the youngest fetal age at which we can and do save premature infants. That suggests confusion in the moral basis of the society – but only for people who think a society can or should have a moral basis. Today we have instead the 'autonomy' of each individual. Postmodern thinkers, at least, celebrate this: we live in an age of 'options' and 'choices', they say; anything goes; there is no moral reason to criticize anyone's choices.

   Consequently, the aborted fetus/ICN patient confusion is not confusion at all. The mother has the choice: is it a mistake in her body or a baby born tragically early? How nice that in our society she can choose either to have it extracted and thrown away or pampered in intensive care! See, autonomy's good for everyone; each person can choose a moral code and live according to it.

Not quite, however. It's true that no one forces a woman to have an abortion. But 'society' does force the premature fetus into intensive care, with possible legal consequences for the mother who resists. And for the mother who does choose abortion, there may be protesters at the abortion clinic and full-page newspaper notices to make her feel guilty. We may honor autonomy, but we aren't yet ready for the society that truly lets everyone be autonomous. We have plenty of remnants that say there is a moral basis to our society. But we're not at all sure what that basis is, nor where it comes from.

In other words, we have, as I suggested above, confusion in the moral basis of our society. We lose the corporate virtues (e.g. compassion) when we claim autonomy, and the remnants of our moral basis only irritate us when they show up as protest groups trying to 'reclaim' morality or as laws made ridiculous by our technology.

Chapter 6 Suffering

1 See Ivan Illich's comments on the difference between pain and suffering in Chapter 3, 'The killing of pain,' in *Medical Nemesis, op.cit.*, p. 133ff.
2 Illich, *ibid.*, p. 134.
3 Illich, *ibid.*, pp. 127–8.
4 'Culture makes pain tolerable by interpreting its necessity; only pain perceived as curable is intolerable.' *Ibid.*, p. 134.
5 Verghese A (1994) *My Own Country: a doctor's story.* Vintage, New York.

Chapter 8 Chronic disease – 1

1 Phillips LS *et al* (2001) Clinical inertia. *Ann Intern Med.* **136**(9): 825–34.
2 Dubos R, *op.cit.*, pp. 198, 199, 207.
3 Kunitz S (1983) *Disease Change and the Role of Medicine: the Navajo experience* University of California Press, pp. 186–7.
4 Mbeki T. www.anc.org.za/ancdocs/history/mbeki/2000/tm0506.html
5 Mbeki T. www.anc.org.za/ancdocs/history/mbeki/2000/tm0709.html
6 Mbeki T. www.gcis.gov.za/media/releases/000914.htm
7 Mbeki T. www.anc.org.za/ancdocs/history/mbeki/2000/tm0709.html

Chapter 9 Treatment

1 Downing R (2000) HIV/AIDS: listen to Mbeki. *Sunday Nation*, November 12, p. 17.
2 Nene ML (2000) Personal communication, November 16.

Chapter 10 Healing

1 The 1965 English title of his first book, published originally in Switzerland in 1940. In the epilogue he refers to World War II, and indeed his first-hand experience of it, as the background for taking a new and more complete look at healing.

2 Arthur Barsky calls this 'the paradox of health,' that in our society 'substantial improvements in health status have not been accompanied by improvements in the subjective feeling of healthiness and physical well-being' (Barsky A (1988) The paradox of health. *NEJM*. **318**(7): 414–18).

3 Keeping costs down was another benefit, but I do not remember it being strongly emphasized in the first decade of family medicine.

4 This negative feedback of our medical system is the main subject of Ivan Illich's 1975 book *Medical Nemesis (op.cit.)*.

Chapter 12 Prevention – 1

1 Dubos R, *Mirage of Health, op.cit.*, pp. 129–30.

2 Thomas McKeown raised a similar set of questions 25 years ago in *The Role of Medicine, op. cit.*, pp. 129–30.

3 Vakil NB and Vaira D (2002) Editorial: medicalisation, limits to medicine, or never enough money to go around? *BMJ*. **324**: 864–5.

Chapter 13 Prevention – 2

1 Nikiforuk A (1991) *The Fourth Horseman: a short history of epidemics, plagues, and other scourges.* Cambridge University Press.

2 Desowitz R (1991) *The Malaria Capers: tales of parasites and people.* Norton, p. 199.

3 World eradication did succeed with smallpox disease in the late 1970s. However, post 9/11 fears have shown the problems of failing to eradicate the virus.

4 'Here I believe it is important to distinguish the role of medicine as an institution from its more limited responsibility for clinical care ... [I]n its larger role, medicine should be concerned with all the influences on health, a conclusion that has considerable bearing on medical education and research as well as on health services.' McKeown T. *The Role Of Medicine, op.cit.*, p. ix.

Chapter 14 Culture

1 Hoebel EA (1966) *Anthropology: the study of man* (3e). McGraw-Hill, p. 71.

2 One of the most poignant and tragic illustrations of this is the story told in Fadiman A (1997) *The Spirit Catches You and You Fall Down.* Farrar, Straus, and Giroux.

3 Stringfellow W (1964) *My People Is The Enemy.* Holt, Rinehart and Winston, New York.

4 Illich, *op.cit.*, p. 39 ff. The *British Medical Journal* revisited this concept in a special issue: April 13, 2002 (vol 324, issue 7342).

Chapter 15 Learning

1 Lundberg D (1984) Exporting doctors to a world in need. *JAMA*. **251**(4): 511–12.

2 H. Jack Geiger's experience, recorded in 'Community-oriented primary healthcare: learning from the Third World' (Chapter 8 of *Global Learning for Health*, edited by Russell Morgan and Bill Rau, NCIH, 1993) is a notable exception dating back to the 1950s and 1960s.

3 Pust RE (1984) US abundance of physicians and international health. *JAMA*. 252(3): 385–8; Hilton D (1991) Medical mission in reverse. *Christianity and Crisis*. September 23, pp. 272–3; Taylor C (1993) Editorial: learning from healthcare experiences in developing countries. *Am J Public Health*. 83(11): 1531–2.

4 Wilson C and Pust R (1999) Preparing health professionals for international health activities: recommended approaches for learning from the developing world. *Educ for Health*. 12(3): 379–87.

5 In 1966, Carl Taylor spoke of a 'continuing exchange and sharing of information' in international health (Ethics for an international health profession. *Science*. 153: 716–20). But the direction of this sharing was clear. He spoke of sharing information 'with foreign colleagues' and admitted that 'there is an uncontrollable tendency for the helping country or organization to draw the recipient country toward its own approach, organizational pattern, and values . . . This should not lead to guilt feelings.' His 1993 *AJPH* article on 'Learning from healthcare experiences in developing countries', noted above, grows logically from this assumption of the 'continuing exchange and sharing of information' though closer to the bilateral exchange Wilson speaks of.

6 Geiger, *op. cit.*

7 Fang HC, Ku YW and Shang TY (1996) The integration of modern and traditional Chinese medicine in the treatment of fractures. a simple method of treatment for fractures of the shafts of both forearm bones. *Clin Orth Rel Res*. 323: 4–111.

8 Kulhara P (1994) Outcome of schizophrenia: some transcultural observations with particular reference to developing countries. *Eur Arch Psychiatr Clin Neurosci*. 244(5): 227–35.

Chapter 16 Poverty

1 Hilfiker D (1996) Scapegoating the poor. *Health Develop*. 3: 3–11.

2 Originally published in *JAMA*, July 8, 1983.

Index